Adolescent Suicide and Self-Injury

Laurel L. Williams • Owen Muir
Editors

Adolescent Suicide and Self-Injury

Mentalizing Theory and Treatment

Springer

Editors
Laurel L. Williams
Menninger Department of Psychiatry and Behavioral Sciences
Baylor College of Medicine
Houston, TX
USA

Owen Muir
Brooklyn Minds Psychiatry
Brooklyn, NY
USA

ISBN 978-3-030-42874-7 ISBN 978-3-030-42875-4 (eBook)
https://doi.org/10.1007/978-3-030-42875-4

This Springer imprint is published by the registered company Springer Nature Switzerland AG
The registered company address is: Gewerbestrasse 11, 6330 Cham, Switzerland

Contents

Contributors

Dickon Bevington Anna Freud National Centre for Children and Families, London, UK

Carl Fleisher Psychiatry and Biobehavioral Sciences, University of California, Los Angeles, Los Angeles, CA, USA

Chris W. Grimes, MSW, LCSW Menninger Department of Psychiatry and Behavioral Sciences, Baylor College of Medicine, Houston, TX, USA

Carlene MacMillan Brooklyn Minds Psychiatry, Brooklyn, NY, USA

Veronica McLaren Department of Psychology, University of Houston, Houston, TX, USA

Owen Muir Brooklyn Minds Psychiatry, Brooklyn, NY, USA

Trudie Rossouw Priory Hospital North London, London, UK

Carla Sharp Department of Psychology, University of Houston, Houston, TX, USA

Laurel L. Williams Menninger Department of Psychiatry and Behavioral Sciences, Baylor College of Medicine, Houston, TX, USA

What Is Mentalizing?

1

Veronica McLaren and Carla Sharp

Introduction

Mentalizing is a deceptively simple concept. In short, to mentalize is to reflect on mental states in oneself and in others [1]. Mentalizing is akin to the concept called Theory of Mind, as in a person's theory about what is in someone's mind. To provide a more practical example of what is meant by this, imagine a friend calls to cancel plans abruptly for the second time in a row. We might first assume that they decided that they don't like us and don't want to see us after all. We might notice that they seem stressed. We could consider that they might have had a rough week and needed a night off. Perhaps an emergency came up and they no longer have time to go out. This example leads to two important observations: First, we notice that we are *uncertain* about the exact intentions behind these actions. This stance of uncertainty is characteristic of mentalizing. Importantly, because we cannot know for sure another's mental state, mentalizing is an inherently *imaginative* activity. Second, mentalizing involves ascribing *intentional* mental states based on cues. This means that when we mentalize, we recognize autonomy. We acknowledge that a person's actions can be explained by their internal state. As we will see, there is quite a bit of complexity to the way we conceptualize mentalizing today. But first it is important to understand how our current understanding came about.

This chapter will discuss the following:

1. Brief history of the term mentalization
2. Understanding of the four dimensions of mentalizing
3. Development of typical mentalizing
4. Importance of parenting and attachment in mentalizing
5. Development of atypical mentalizing

V. McLaren · C. Sharp (✉)
Department of Psychology, University of Houston, Houston, TX, USA
e-mail: vjmclaren@uh.edu; csharp2@uh.edu

L. L. Williams, O. Muir (eds.), *Adolescent Suicide and Self-Injury*,
https://doi.org/10.1007/978-3-030-42875-4_1

Brief History

The term "mentalize" was first recorded in writing in 1807 and made it into the *Oxford English Dictionary* in 1906. In the 1960s, the concept of mentalizing was brought into the psychological world by psychoanalytic theorists. Freud's concepts of *binding* and *physical working out* set the stage for the appearance of mentalization [2]. These concepts involve "the transformation of physical quantity into psychical quality" and "the setting up of associative pathways" [3]—in other words, turning something physical (i.e., an observed cue) into something psychological (i.e., a mental state). The word *mentalization* first appeared in the psychological literature in the writings of French psychoanalysts [4]. In 1997, Lecours and Bouchard developed a model for mentalization based on this tradition.

In the 1980s, the term "Theory of Mind" (ToM) gained traction in the psychological realm. When coined by primatologists Premack and Woodruff, ToM was described as an individual's ability to attribute mental states to themselves and to others [5]. This coining was prompted by the discovery that chimpanzees can in fact infer the mental states of humans; when presented with a human struggling with a problem and given several photographs, one of which contained a solution to the problem, the chimpanzees consistently chose the correct photograph. In essence, in order to choose the correct solution, the chimpanzees had to recognize the intentions of the other. Shortly thereafter, work on ToM began in humans.

Much work on ToM in humans has been based on the concept of false belief. In short, a scenario is presented to a subject in which a character comes to believe something that the subject knows to be false. In order to arrive at the correct conclusions about the character's beliefs, the subject must be able to decouple mental states from reality. In other words, they must recognize that what is in their mind is not the same as what as in the minds of others. A wide range of research using this sort of task has revealed that we are not born with this understanding; rather, this ability develops between ages three and four [6]. Thus far, we have only looked at ToM as it develops naturally; studying the impact of nurture on mentalizing brought it into the realm of attachment.

Mentalization, as it is used in mentalization-based treatment (MBT), developed when it was adopted by attachment theorists. Fonagy found that infant attachment could be predicted by a parent's "predisposition to see relationships in terms of mental content" [7]. In other words, the better a parent could mentalize their baby's mind, the more likely the child was to have secure attachment. These findings sparked a boom of literature related to mentalizing, beginning in the 1990s, resulting in more than 4000 scientific studies published on the topic by 2014 [8]. Since then, mentalization has been studied developmentally [9], biologically [10], and even musically [11]. In particular, neuroscience has made major contributions to our understanding of mentalizing. In addition to providing support for the importance of attachment in mentalizing capacity, neuroscientific studies have identified dissociable neural networks for mentalizing [8]. This means that not only is mentalizing an observable phenomenon via neural activity, but also we now know through brain sciences the distinct dimensions underlying the capacity to mentalize (see the section on The Four Dimensions).

As evidenced by its rich history, mentalizing encompasses diverse approaches and facets. It becomes necessary to have an organized understanding of how the process of mentalizing can be broken down. Thus, four dimensions of mentalization have been identified—corresponding to the previously mentioned dissociable neural networks—which give meaning to particular instances of mentalization.

The Four Dimensions

The definition of mentalizing we gave earlier leaves many questions unanswered. We might think of the dimensions—or, as Fonagy and Bateman would have it, "polarities" (Fig. 1.1)—of mentalizing as the answers to questions we could ask about a particular instance of mentalizing. Recall that any instance of mentalizing represents a reflection on the mental states in oneself or others. The first question we might ask is:

Whose Mental State? Self Versus Other

The self versus other dimension is just what it seems: it refers to whether the mental state being considered is in *oneself* or in *another*. Despite its apparent simplicity, it is not especially easy in practice. Consider from the beginning of the chapter our friend who has just canceled plans with us. If you go back and read everything we considered about the situation, you will find that none of them related to our own mental state. We often neglect to consider our own mental state because we assume that we already know it; however, in the same way that we cannot know the contents of someone else's mind, the contents of our own minds are not as available to us as we might think.

Fig. 1.1 Polarities

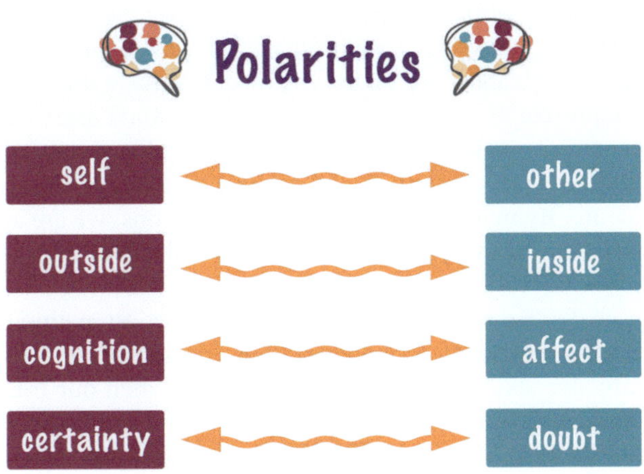

This is not to say that mentalizing the self is always the challenge. We might just as easily have focused only on our own mental states—we are hurt; we were looking forward to the night out; we are mad that we wasted all that time planning for the outing; we wanted to be better friends with this person. The challenge is finding the balance between mentalizing self and other, and arriving at an integrated understanding of how they interact with one another. When it comes to the self–other polarity, it is really the ability to move smoothly back and forth between these perspectives that is characteristic of good mentalizing. Getting stuck on one perspective, either self or other, is a characteristic of poor mentalizing. When you ask a youth arguing about your intentions "What were you thinking?" and the answer is "I don't know!" this is self–other mentalizing that is stuck and thus leading to characteristic difficulties.

Once we know whose mental state we are talking about, the next important question we might ask is:

What Kind of Mental State? Affective Versus Cognitive

Affective versus cognitive refers to the nature of the mental state. *Affective* mentalizing is of feelings, while *cognitive* mentalizing is of thoughts. This distinction refers to not only the characteristics of the mental state we consider for an individual, but also the nature of our understanding of the mental state. Thus, affective mentalizing is more similar to empathy or emotional contagion, while cognitive mentalizing is rooted in reasoning and perspective-taking. This distinction is made clear in the differences between the Theory of Mind Mechanism and the Empathizing System [12].

The Theory of Mind Mechanism corresponds to cognitive mentalizing and processes metarepresentations, or M-representations. M-representations were defined by Alan Leslie as consisting of an agent, an information relation, and an expression [13]. Baron-Cohen redefines these elements as an agent, an attitude, and a proposition [12]—in other words, a person, a type of mental state (e.g., believes, thinks, wants), and the content of that mental state. For example, when we consider our friend who canceled on us, we might create the M-representation "Our friend does not know that I went out of my way to plan for our outing" or "Our friend wanted to cancel our plans when we first made them." Importantly, each of these is a representation of what is in our friend's mind and thus a representation of a representation—a metarepresentation. Although we might not always recognize that these are representations and not reality, they are in fact always representational in nature. By making use of metarepresentations, we are able to denote that something is not necessarily real, but that we think it may be—decoupling the mind from physical reality.

Affective mentalizing corresponds to the Empathizing System, which processes E-representations. E-representations consist of the self, an affective state, and an affective state proposition. For example, when our friend cancels on us, we might notice that they are stressed and create the E-representation "We are sorry that they are stressed." While an M-representation might contain an emotion ("We see that our friend is stressed"), it does not include an impact of the emotion on the self. This means that a representation regarding an emotion is only an E-representation when the affective state has an effect on the self. Similarly, an instance of mentalizing regarding an emotion is only affective mentalizing when the emotion impacts the self; thus, affective mentalizing is quite similar to empathy.

Now that we understand the kind of mental state we are working with, we might wonder:

What Kind of Cues Are Used? Internal Versus External

When we mentalize, we must base our representation on something. The internal versus external dimension refers to the nature of the cues that are used to inform the representation of a mental state. Mentalizing might be based on observable features, meaning the things a person says or does—this would denote mentalization of external features. These can be things like facial expression, tone of voice, or even the words that are used. When we notice that our friend seems stressed, we likely use external cues. Perhaps their voice sounds rushed, or perhaps they say, "Things have been crazy this week."

In contrast, mentalizing that is based on internal cues relies on an understanding of internal experiences, such as thoughts and feelings. Internal mentalizing requires an initial hypothesis. For example, once we notice that our friend is stressed, we are able to use internal mentalizing to go deeper. Based on the external cue that their tone of voice sounds stressed, we might now think things like "They wish they could hang out with us but they don't have the time."

Now that we have answered all of those questions, we might still be wondering how it all comes together. The final question we ask is:

How Does the Awareness Come About? Automatic Versus Controlled

Perhaps the most important dimension to consider is automatic versus controlled—alternatively called the implicit versus explicit dimension. This is the polarity we are trying to "lubricate" the most with MBT, to allow the kids and families we are working with to be able to transition deftly from implicit mentalizing to slower, more controlled, and more explicit mentalizing that allows them to understand their way out of a misunderstanding!

Automatic, or implicit, mentalizing happens when we are not thinking about it. You might think of it as your intuition. In automatic mentalizing, multiple cues are processed simultaneously; thus, automatic mentalizing is fast and does not require attention or effort [14]. In order to process so much information so quickly, we rely on heuristics, or mental shortcuts. If you were to think deeply about the inner worlds of every stranger you passed on the street, you would barely make it a block without mental exhaustion! It is important to have heuristics to save time and energy as we go through our day in a sea of minds—most of which don't actually matter to us! These heuristics are learned through exposure and repetition; when a certain event has the same outcome over and over, our brains come to expect that outcome once the event occurs. When things go smoothly, automatic mentalizing is sufficient; thus, most day-to-day mentalizing is automatic [15]. For example, if our friend had not canceled on us and we had gotten to see them as we had planned, we would likely not have thought about their motivation. Instead, we would have trusted our intuition to interpret their thoughts and feelings. However, in the unexpected situation where our friend cancels on us, relying on our intuition gets us in trouble. Recall that our first thought was that they didn't want to see us in the first place. Even though there is no reason for us to think this, our mental heuristics have pieced together an explanation based on cognitive biases. This does not seem to be a good strategy for the situation. What might we have done instead?

When something out of the ordinary happens, good mentalizers can shift to controlled, or explicit, mentalizing. Controlled mentalizing is a much slower and deliberate process. In contrast to automatic mentalizing, controlled mentalizing requires that things be processed one at a time [14]. Just like it sounds, we are in control of this process; thus, it requires attention, effort, and intention. For example, when our friend cancels on us, we can slow down and acknowledge that we feel hurt but recognize that we don't know what is inside their mind. We then can share these concerns and ask them for clarification. When we do this, we have changed not only the way we interpret the situation, but also the way we interact with it. It is clear that in this situation, controlled mentalizing is necessary, while using automatic mentalizing gets us in trouble. However, using controlled mentalizing when the situation does not call for it can also be bad. Let us return to the situation in which we ended up on this outing with our friend. If we are stopping to think the whole time about what they think of us or whether they are having a good time, we waste mental energy on working through these thoughts rather than enjoying our time with our friend. We are also likely making our friend feel awkward, as if they are under a magnifying glass or as if we don't trust them. This kind of overthinking is called *hypermentalizing* and can be counterproductive in most interactions, as it leads to overattribution of mental states beyond what there is evidence for [16].

We can see that neither implicit nor explicit mentalizing is inherently indicative of bad mentalizing, but a good mentalizer is one who can identify which is appropriate for the situation. Next, we will examine how our mentalizing ability develops and the things that contribute to making us good mentalizers.

The Development of Typical Mentalizing

Although mentalizing is a seemingly natural process, we are not born with an understanding of the mind. Kim [17] compares this concept to our linguistic ability; just as we are not born knowing language but are equipped to acquire it, given sufficient input, we seem to be equipped to learn to mentalize, given enough exposure to mental states. In this section, we will discuss the acquisition of our mentalizing ability, first by examining the normative timeline of mentalizing development and then by looking at the processes by which we are exposed to the mind and that promote this successful development of mentalizing ability.

The Normative Timeline

Development of mentalizing ability is generally organized into four stages. Each stage is marked by the acquisition of a new mentalizing-related ability and is thus characterized by distinct ways of thinking about mental states. We will survey each of these four stages and the associated mentalizing capabilities, beginning with infancy.

Infancy Infancy, encompassing birth to age one, is characterized by the development of what is known as teleological thinking. This teleological stance refers to the rational construal of perceived actions; in other words, infants come to expect others' actions to be directed at achieving a goal in the most efficient way possible, within the constraints of reality [18]. In teleological thinking, everything is constrained to the physical realm and mental states are not yet considered; goals and actions taken to achieve those goals consist only of things that are directly observable. Thus, over the first year of life, the infant comes to understand that actions are goal directed and they expect others to act rationally given their goals. In this way, the infant can, without any understanding of unobservable mental states, make sense of current actions and make predictions about future actions [17].

Infants also begin to recognize themselves as teleological agents, both physically and socially. In other words, they learn that their actions can bring about changes in the physical world, like making a ball move, and the social world, like when smiling at Mom leads to Mom smiling back [1]. This allows the infant to begin to develop a foundation for later emotional understanding.

Toddlerhood During toddlerhood, which encompasses ages two and three, the child develops what is called the intentional stance. In contrast to the teleological stance, the intentional stance recognizes that actions are caused by prior unobservable states of mind [19]. This is the first hint of attention to mental states; in this stage, children can understand goals and actions in a more mentalistic frame. They can conceptualize things like desires, wants, and intentions [20]. Further, children begin to develop an understanding of emotions and a capacity for empathy. The toddler's empathy and other mentalizing instances are all considered to consist only of implicit mentalizing, as explicit mentalizing has not yet developed [17].

Importantly, the child's thinking during toddlerhood is marked by psychic equivalence. Psychic equivalence is the lack of a separation between mental states and reality, or the idea that what is in the child's mind is real. This is especially apparent in the pretend play characteristic of this age group. Toddlers' pretend play can feel very real and they can get lost in magical thinking, like the child who believes there is a monster under the bed. Thus, while the toddler can now conceptualize mental states, the separation between internal and external events is still blurred.

Early childhood In early childhood, children aged four and five begin understanding that actions result from beliefs. This is accompanied by the monumental achievement of passing the false-belief task, described earlier in the chapter. Passing this task requires the use of explicit mentalizing as well as the separation of mental states from reality. This means that in early childhood, children are able to deliberately and consciously consider mental states and can fully understand that reality does not necessarily correspond with the said mental states. With this decoupling comes the ability to deceive, tell jokes, and play tricks [21].

Further, the child can now grasp the idea that mental states are transient and that action is informed both by these transient states and by stable characteristics [22]. In other words, temporary mental states like thoughts and emotions interact with permanent traits like personality to inform behavior. These ideas provide the foundation for an emerging sense of identity.

Middle childhood Middle childhood comprises ages six to eleven and gives way to more complex mentalizing abilities. In this age range, children can organize their memories into a causal–temporal framework [23]. This means they can begin forming narrative, autobiographical understandings of themselves and their experiences, leading to a coherent and consistent self across time, although at this stage these ideas are still rather concrete and unintegrated. Children also gain higher-order mentalizing abilities—an ability to think about what one person thinks is in another person's mind—and the ability to consider mixed emotions. Despite these important gains, children in this stage still lack authenticity when talking about mental states. This lack of authenticity is referred to as *pretend mode* and is due to a developing sense of morality and societal values; mental state reasoning is heavily influenced by ideas about what one *should* think and feel. Nevertheless, the gains made in middle childhood pave the way for identity consolidation and social thinking in adolescence.

Adolescence Adolescence is characterized by incredible expansion of the social world as well as the social brain. Not only are adolescents' brains equipped for sophisticated and complicated perspective-taking, but also their interest and capacity for novelty-seeking experiences expands. This is necessary for them to become autonomous; however, the increased reward and amygdala sensitivity underlying this expansion is not matched with increased prefrontal cortex development and adolescents continue to need the support of caregivers to scaffold the development of mentalizing abilities. An important aspect during this period is the beginning of the development of mature self-reflective capacities. Adolescents begin to mentalize the self in a very active way and are charged with integrating multiple self-hypotheses with feedback from parents, peers, teachers, and the environment. They are now beginning the process of consolidating their identities. This is a complex task, and it does not go equally smoothly for all adolescents. It is therefore no surprise that adolescence is the developmental period of onset for most psychiatric disorders, particularly personality disorders, which are of course highly associated with self-harm and suicidality—the foci of this book.

The Importance of Parenting and Attachment

As stated previously, although we are equipped (hard wired) to learn to mentalize, we are not born knowing how. In order to become true mentalizers, we must be taught. Thus, the development of mentalizing is hugely reliant on caregiving and, in particular, attachment. In this section, we will examine the relationship between caregiving, attachment, and mentalizing more closely, and see how the interplay between the three fosters one's own mentalizing ability.

Emotion regulation As we have just discussed, in infancy children are unable to understand internal states and rely solely on external stimuli to construct an understanding of the world. This includes their own emotional states. They are thus reliant on the outside world to help them make sense of emotions. Parents are vital to this understanding by way of affect mirroring; when a parent notices a child's distress, the parent is naturally inclined to mirror the affect in order to soothe or downregulate the infant's arousal [24]. This is called *marked mirroring*. In order for marked mirroring to be successful, it must have two vital characteristics.

First, a caregiver's response must be congruent with the internal state of the infant. The parent's ability to create a congruent affect is largely dependent on their own mentalizing ability. The mental state of the infant must be correctly identified in order to create a response that matches. This requires the parent to accurately mentalize the child. If identified incorrectly and internalized by the infant, the cue will lead to a fragmented sense of self known as the *alien self* (which is discussed further in the following section). As a brief example, if a child is crying, a congruent response would be the mother making a sad face.

Second, the response must be marked; the parent must indicate that the emotion is not their own but that they are aware of the baby's internal states. This is done by modifying the emotion such that it is distinguishable from the parent's own affect. For example, a parent may mix the congruent emotion with an incongruent one, such as concern, or they might exaggerate or slow down the emotional expression. In any case, in order to present a marked response, the parent must be able to regulate their own emotions. If the parent is unable to modify the emotion and instead becomes distressed themselves, the infant learns that their own negative internal experiences have negative consequences in the external world and are dangerous. The sad face from the prior example would have to be a bit exaggerated to be marked; for the sad child's crying to be met with the mother's own weeping is congruent but not at all marked and doesn't allow for self-other differentiation.

When a caregiver's response is both marked and congruent, it both teaches the infant to associate this representation with their emotional state and helps to regulate the emotion [25]. Thus, the mirroring not only helps the infant learn to recognize emotions but also lays the foundation for emotional self-regulation.

Pedagogical interactions We must rely on ostensive cueing when it comes to learning about emotions. Ostensive cueing signals to the child that the adult is about to communicate something that is worth learning. Because observational learning alone is not sufficient, we cannot learn by observing what emotions feel like; we must instead trust our caregivers to teach us. Similarly, when we are learning to mentalize, we cannot simply observe the internal states of others; we must be taught. These teaching interactions, including ostensive cueing, are known as pedagogical interactions, and they require a pedagogical stance—one that is receptive to and trusting of new information—to be successful [26]. This stance starts with the adult; the adult must first mentalize the child to understand what the infant knows and does not know, be receptive to the infant's needs to recognize that there is some new piece of information that ought to be taught, and finally signal to the infant their intent to convey some information to them. The infant then adopts the pedagogical stance themselves—receptive, attentive, and ready to be taught.

As is clear from the mere preparation for a teaching moment, this stance is costly for the adult. Thus, it requires the good intent of the teacher, a characteristic that often leads to secure attachment. Secure attachment is associated with the belief on the infant's part that the information given by the caregiver is trustworthy. This is known as epistemic trust—that is to say, trust in social information. When the infant can trust the parent, they are not on their own in coming to an understanding of the world; they can instead rely on the parent to guide them.

Attachment security We have already seen two specific ways in which parenting fosters mentalizing ability. We will now examine the complex relationship between parental attachment and mentalizing and child attachment and mentalizing. Recall from earlier in this chapter the study by Fonagy that first prompted attachment theorists' interest in mentalizing; parental mentalization was found to affect attachment as early as infancy [7]. To understand this relationship and how it leads to child mentalizing ability, we must first go back to parental attachment.

When a parent is securely attached, they are capable of mentalizing themselves and their children. These highly mentalistic interactions provide a secure base for the child and foster secure attachment. As previously noted, this secure attachment leads to epistemic trust and makes the child open to learning via pedagogical communication. Thus, the parent who is a competent mentalizer can now teach the child to become a competent mentalizer themselves.

We can see how much must be in place for mentalizing to develop successfully. We will turn now to discussing what can happen to one's mentalizing ability and in turn one's mental health when these things are not in place.

The Development of Atypical Mentalizing

We have just seen how important caregiver attachment and mentalizing is for the development of mentalizing. What happens when these things are not in place? The insecurely attached parent will be unable to accurately mentalize the child. Failed caregiver mentalizing—that is to say, fewer than 30% of responses being contingent—leads to attachment trauma [27]. In its most extreme form, generally when caregivers are abusive, this trauma manifests as disorganized attachment,

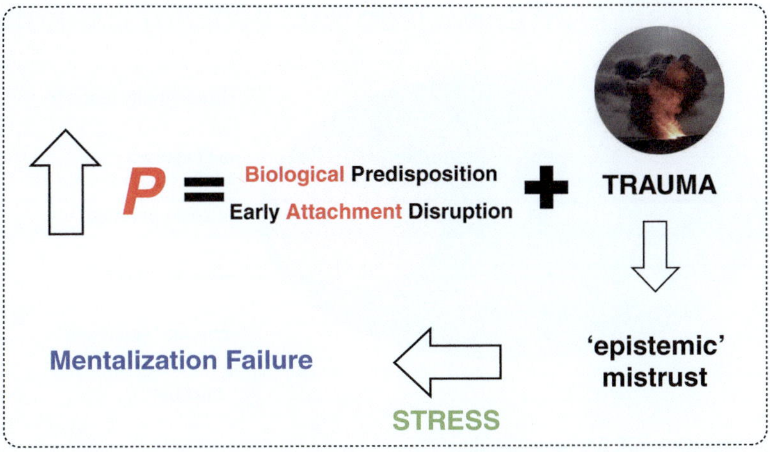

Fig. 1.2 Mentalization-based treatment (MBT) understanding. *P* general psychopathology factor

where the child is unable to develop any consistent strategy for relating to the caregiver [28]. Attachment trauma dismantles epistemic trust—the child does not believe that information from others, or even from their own experience, is to be trusted—leaving the child without a pathway to learning vital information about the world and the mind [29]. Thus, attachment trauma not only increases the child's distress as they are faced with maltreatment, but also keeps them from developing the ability to regulate their emotions, which might enable them to cope with maltreatment [30]. As a result, the child withdraws from the mental world [25]. The consequences of this can be very serious and pervasive. In fact, it is exactly this breakdown in social learning that has led to the problems that inspired the writing of this book (Fig. 1.2).

The Alien Self

When attachment is disorganized, the child cannot integrate their emotional awareness with their sense of how they are organized in their minds [31]. This is best illustrated through incongruent mirroring. As previously discussed, when a caregiver provides the child with an incongruent cue and the child internalizes that cue, an *alien self* (Fig. 1.3) is created for the child wherein mental states are incongruent with the external experience. This alien self sounds like a wonky concept, but perhaps if it is conceptualized as your "mistrustful emotional press secretary" feeding you bad information, we can understand how problematic it can be. A friend saying, "You look great in that dress" would elicit a response from our alien self along the lines of "Why are they LYING to me?!" This is thought to undermine the sense of self. It has been suggested that suicide and self-harm represent "the fantasized destruction of this alien other within the self," especially in people with borderline personality

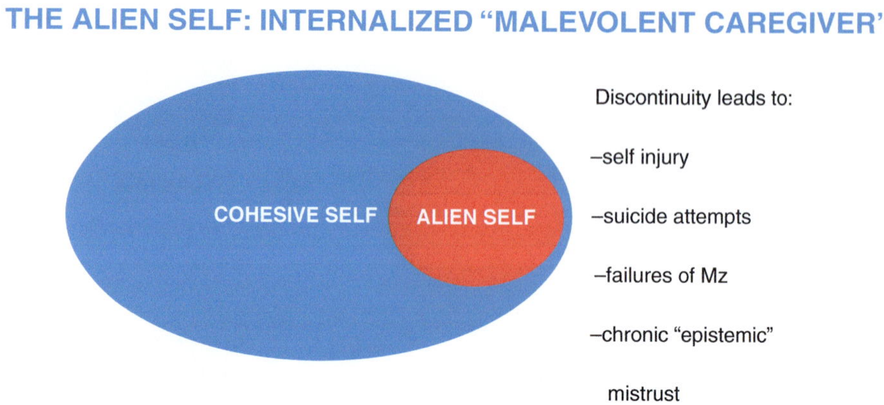

Fig. 1.3 The alien self. *Mz* mentalization

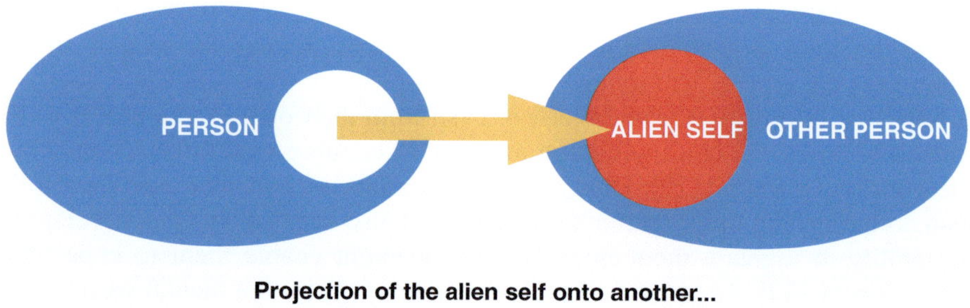

Fig. 1.4 Externalization of the alien self

disorder [32]. However, in an environment in which one cannot and should not trust the good intentions of their caregivers—they will hurt you!—that alien self could come in quite useful. "Be extra careful," it constantly whispers, "no one is to be trusted!" Thus, when we grow up with danger and maltreatment, this alien self is actually very correct but very hard to live with (Fig. 1.4)

Pre-mentalizing Modes: The Target of Treatment

When mentalizing development is disrupted, attempts at mentalizing will be stuck in one of the three pre-mentalizing modes. You will recognize these modes from our discussion of the normative timeline; each is an important part of the development of complete mentalizing ability. However, when there is a disruption in the developmental process, like a trauma or attachment disruption, these modes can persist or re-emerge in adulthood.

Psychic equivalence Like the toddler who cannot separate fantasy from reality, an individual with attachment disruption may use psychic equivalence. In older individuals, this blurring of internal and external experience could be simply the conviction that they know exactly what someone else is thinking or feeling, or it could be the fear associated with a posttraumatic flashback. In both cases, what is in the mind is experienced as real or as necessarily true. As a result, the subjective experience becomes too real because any subjective possibility feels like objective reality.

Pretend mode While internal and external states are blurred in psychic equivalence, the two are kept completely separate in pretend mode. Just as the older child is unable to fully integrate the two and mentalize authentically, the traumatized adult may be able to talk about mental states based on what one *should* be feeling. While this might result in apparent competence, there will be a lack of a fully authentic connection with mental states, as they are, in fact, using rational and intellectual processes devoid of any affect [33]. As a result, the mental state is decoupled from the affect, keeping it separate from the rest of the mental world, and the individual becomes detached and isolated [34]. This is especially evident in dissociative experiences [31].

Teleological mode In the teleological mode, infants are not yet able to conceive of mental states. An individual with attachment trauma may exhibit the same sort of ignorance of mental states. In this mode, the traumatized adult will equate others' desires and feelings with observable behavior. This might mean requiring a physical action for proof of a subjective state—for example, the idea that one can only be loved if one is physically touched [35]. Similarly, an individual might believe that physical acts are the only way to express their own internal experience for others to understand it.

Conclusion

Our goal in this chapter has been to provide an accessible definition of the construct of mentalizing to lay the foundation for the rest of the chapters in this book. In conclusion, we would like to emphasize a few points specifically related to self-harm and suicidality in adolescents—the focus of this book. We have discussed how mentalizing is an imaginative activity during which we adopt a stance of curiosity and uncertainty about the contents of others' minds and our own. In contrast, self-harm may be seen as teleological—making use of a concrete action to manage intolerable and intensely painful mental states. Similarly, suicidal ideation is about wanting to engage in physical action to end intense psychic pain, and a suicide attempt is the only option to signal and express a desperate psychological need for connectedness. These are all non-mentalizing behaviors that avoid reflection on and engagement with the mind. In the chapters that follow, we will see how mentalizing is restored in young people who have lost the capacity to use their reflective capacities to manage intense psychological pain.

References

1. Allen J, Fonagy P, Bateman AW. Mentalizing in clinical practice. Washington, DC: American Psychiatric Publishing; 2008.
2. Lecours S, Bouchard M-A. Dimensions of mentalisation: outlining levels of psychic transformation. Int J Psychoanal. 1997;78(1997):855–75.
3. Laplanche J, Pontalis JB. The language of psycho-analysis (trans: Nicholson-Smith D). Oxford: Norton; 1973. pp. xv, 510.
4. Marty P, M'Uzan D. La pensée opératoire. Rev Francaise Pschanalyse. 1963;27:1345–56.
5. Premack D, Woodruff G. Does the chimpanzee have a theory of mind? Behav Brain Sci. 1978;1(4):515–26.
6. Wellman HM, Cross D, Watson J. Meta-analysis of theory-of-mind development: the truth about false belief. Child Dev. 2001;72(3):655–84.
7. Fonagy P, Steele M, Steele H, Moran GS, Higgitt AC. The capacity for understanding mental states: the reflective self in parent and child and its significance for security of attachment. Infant Ment Health J. 1991;12(3):201–18.
8. Luyten P, Fonagy P. The neurobiology of mentalizing. Personal Disord Theory Res Treat. 2015;6(4):366–79.
9. Fonagy P, Luyten P. A developmental, mentalization-based approach to the understanding and treatment of borderline personality disorder. Dev Psychopathol. 2009;21(4):1355–81.
10. Mitkovic V, Pejovic M, Mandic M, Lecic T. Timeline of intergenerational child maltreatment: the mind–brain–body interplay. Curr Psychiatry Rep. 2017;19(8):50.
11. Downey L, Blezat A, Nicholas J, Omar R, Golden H, Mahoney C, et al. Mentalising music in frontotemporal dementia. Cortex. 2013;49(7):1844–55.
12. Baron-Cohen S, Golan O, Chakrabarti B, Belmonte MK. Social cognition and autism spectrum conditions. In: Sharp C, Fonagy P, Goodyer I, editors. Social cognition and developmental psychopathology. Oxford: Oxford University Press; 2008. p. 39.
13. Leslie AM. Pretense and representation: the origins of "theory of mind". Psychol Rev. 1987;94(4):15.
14. Satpute AB, Lieberman MD. Integrating automatic and controlled processes into neurocognitive models of social cognition. Brain Res. 2006;1079(1):86–97.
15. Fonagy P, Bateman AW, Luyten P. Introduction and overview. In: Bateman AW, Fonagy P, editors. Handbook of mentalizing in mental health practice. Washington, DC: American Psychiatric Publishing; 2012.
16. Sharp C, Ha C, Carbone C, Kim S, Perry K, Williams L, et al. Hypermentalizing in adolescent inpatients: treatment effects and association with borderline traits. J Personal Disord. 2013;27(1):3–18.
17. Kim S. The mind in the making: developmental and neurobiological origins of mentalizing. Personal Disord Theory Res Treat. 2015;6(4):356–65.
18. Gergely G, Csibra G. Teleological reasoning in infancy: the naïve theory of rational action. Trends Cogn Sci. 2003;7(7):287–92.
19. Wellman HM, Phillips A. Developing intentional understandings. In: Malle BF, Moses LJ, Baldwin DA, editors. Intentions and intentionality: foundations of social cognition. Cambridge: MIT Press; 2000.
20. Wellman HM, Lagattuta KH. Developing understandings of mind. In: Baron-Cohen S, Tager-Flusberg H, Cohen DJ, editors. Understanding other minds: perspectives from developmental cognitive neuroscience. 2nd ed. New York: Oxford University Press; 2000. p. 21–49.
21. Sodian B, Taylor C, Harris PL, Perner J. Early deception and the child's theory of mind: false trails and genuine markers. Child Dev. 1991;62(3):468–83.
22. Fonagy P, Allison E. What is mentalization? The concept and its foundations in developmental research. In: Midgley N, Vrouva J, editors. Minding the child: mentalization-based interventions with children, young people and their families. Hove: Routledge; 2012. p. 11–53.

23. Povinelli DJ, Eddy T. The unduplicated self. In: Rochat P, editor. The self in infancy: theory and research. Amsterdam: Elsevier; 1995. p. 7.
24. Kim S, Fonagy P, Allen J, Martinez S, Iyengar U, Strathearn L. Mothers who are securely attached in pregnancy show more attuned infant mirroring 7 months postpartum. Infant Behav Dev. 2014;37(4):491–504.
25. Fonagy P, Gergely G, Target M. The parent–infant dyad and the construction of the subjective self. J Child Psychol Psychiatry. 2007;48(3–4):288–328.
26. Gergely G, Egyed K, Király I. On pedagogy. Dev Sci. 2007;10(1):139–46.
27. Allen J. Mentalizing in the development and treatment of attachment trauma. London: Karmac; 2013.
28. Main M, Solomon J. Procedures for identifying infants as disorganized/disoriented during the Ainsworth Strange Situation. In: Greenberg T, Cicchetti D, Cummings EM, editors. Attachment in the preschool years: theory, research, and intervention. Chicago: University of Chicago Press; 1990.
29. Fonagy P, Allison E. The role of mentalizing and epistemic trust in the therapeutic relationship. Psychotherapy. 2014;51(3):372–80.
30. Fonagy P, Target M. Early intervention and the development of self-regulation. Psychoanal Inq. 2002;22(3):307–35.
31. Fonagy P. The mentalization-focused approach to social development. In: Allen JG, Fonagy P, editors. The handbook of mentalization-based treatment. Chichester: Wiley; 2006. p. 53–99.
32. Fonagy P. Attachment and borderline personality disorder. J Am Psychoanal Assoc. 1998;48(4):1129–46.
33. Bateman A, Fonagy P. Mentalization-based treatment. Psychoanal Inq. 2013;33(6):595–613.
34. Bateman A, Fonagy P. Mentalization-based treatment of BPD. J Personal Disord. 2004;18(1):36–51.
35. Fonagy P, Bateman AW. Mechanisms of change in mentalization-based treatment of BPD. J Clin Psychol. 2006;62(4):411–30.

Core Mentalizing Techniques

2

Laurel L. Williams

Introduction

In this chapter, we will introduce the specific techniques involved in developing a mentalizing approach to therapy. As we discussed in Chap. 1, one of the best things about mentalizing therapy is that you, dear reader, already know how to mentalize. You do this every day and, most likely, your patients mentalize in their everyday lives as well. Our goal in this chapter is to lay out, step by step, the mechanics of mentalizing more purposefully and in a "metacognitive" manner. By this, we mean that not only are you assisting your patient to mentalize but also you are simultaneously observing how the relationships between you and the patient are able to foster mentalization. That is to say, you will simultaneously maintain a "curious" bird's-eye view of the session while working in therapy.

To that end, we have five specific core mentalizing techniques to learn in this chapter:

1. The mentalizing stance
2. Appropriately engaging when in psychic equivalence mode
3. Appropriately engaging when in teleological mode
4. Appropriately engaging when in pretend mode
5. The mentalizing loop (or notice and name)

L. L. Williams (✉)
Menninger Department of Psychiatry and Behavioral Sciences, Baylor College of Medicine, Houston, TX, USA
e-mail: laurelw@bcm.edu

L. L. Williams, O. Muir (eds.), *Adolescent Suicide and Self-Injury*,
https://doi.org/10.1007/978-3-030-42875-4_2

The Mentalizing Stance

The mentalizing stance is the steady base on which the other techniques will rely. In our review of the theory behind mentalizing in Chap. 1, we discussed the concept of building epistemic trust through the activation of the attachment system. The mentalizing stance is how this happens in practice. It cannot be overstated that without the mentalizing stance, there is little chance for mentalizing to develop or be maintained!

In mentalization-based treatment (MBT), we use the concept that the stance is a table with four legs. Without each of the legs, the stance becomes unsteady and prone to breakdown. Much of what is involved in the stance will feel familiar to therapists regardless of their approach, and that too is by design. We have noted that mentalizing is a necessary human trait that allows us to activate epistemic trust and develop meaningful relationships. However, for various reasons, a therapist can be knocked off balance from the stance and, as a result, find the session is knocked off balance as well. If, in challenging sessions, you can manage to keep your focus on re-engaging the stance, it can lead to more helpful therapy for your patients.

Why is the stance prone to being knocked off balance? Simply put, it is because throughout the day, mentalizing is *normally* turned on and off. As we noted in Chap. 1, humans—including therapists—are not meant to constantly *explicitly* mentalize. Being tired, hungry, or preoccupied with the tasks of the day [like completing the necessary elements of an intake appointment or reading this book]—or believing you already know what you or others think—turns off explicit mentalizing. Even the activation of the attachment system itself can TURN OFF mentalizing! For example, if your attachment system is activated, you may not closely examine the thoughts and feelings of the person who has activated your attachment (i.e., consider the proverb "Love is blind" as you ponder how attachment activation turns off mentalizing). However, therapy sessions aren't meant to be ordinary conversations after all, and so, as a therapist, your goal in MBT is focusing on the presence or absence of mentalizing. That's it. No insights or skills need to be used beyond keeping an observing mind for the presence or absence of mentalizing! This is the first step in maintaining an inherently unsteady mentalizing stance (Fig. 2.1).

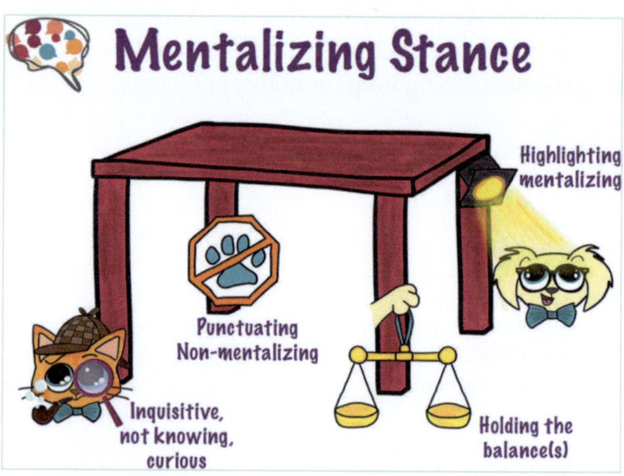

Fig. 2.1 The mentalizing stance

1. Inquisitive "not knowing" stance
2. Holding the balance
3. Stopping non-mentalizing
4. Highlighting and reinforcing active mentalizing

While the four legs are listed above in numerical order, in a session, you would not be moving between them in a rote or robotic fashion. The stance is more that you should see yourself as consciously attending to these elements, such that if one is missing or wobbling, you would make efforts to re-engage that aspect of the stance. MBT therapists physically exhibit this even in the manner in which they sit while in a session—literally on "the edge of their seat." This is because MBT is a very active therapy. Sitting back while occasionally uttering "Go on" or "Tell me more" is unlikely to foster mentalization.

"Not Knowing"

Being fundamentally inquisitive or "not knowing" is perhaps closest to a state of perpetual curiosity. On the surface, being curious sounds fairly basic and, to be fair, it is. However, consider your most recent therapy session: how quickly did you move from a curious approach to mentally preparing your next step in telling the patient something about themselves, the process, or the outcome? Staying curious can be a challenge—especially if you as the therapist believe *you already know* something your patient doesn't. In other words, having a GREAT IDEA that they "just" haven't figured out yet is the opposite of "not knowing."

Let's take a moment here to point out a specific word in the previous paragraph: "just." Since MBT therapy is about allowing families to take a curious stance using language as the immunization against impulsivity and self-harm, it makes sense that we will pay attention to the words we use. Some words are so reliably non-mentalized that we can draw attention to their intrusion to stop subsequent non-mentalized ideas in their tracks. As you attune your listening to the patient (and yourself), consider how there are many words that can cut off mentalizing and quickly move the session out of a curious stance. As our first goal in the stance is to maintain curiosity, we encourage therapists to consider how they may respond to hearing the words and phrases listed below and help reconnect from these MBT "swear words" back to a more curious stance. One example has a therapist using their fingers as antennae that slowly rise up from their head when one of these words or phrases is used. The goal here is not to shame a person's language choice but more to assist everyone to really pay close attention to what is said and what might be meant. Here is a short list of words we call out in sessions as "four-letter words" in MBT. We imagine that you, dear reader, can likely think of many more that convey a dismissive or non-curious stance.

1. Just: There is no other explanation for what I'm saying.
2. Always: Is this "always" true? That seems extreme.
3. Never: This is the same as "always."

4. Must: I know how you MUST feel because I'm psychic.
5. But: This words says "Sure, I just said something nice, but it was a lie and now I will invalidate it." See, the word does the same thing even in the previous sentence!
6. Totally understand: In many situations when this phrase is used, there is likely evidence that the person does not.
7. Look: You are clearly too dumb to understand, so I will make my point again without taking your perspective into account.
8. I hear you: This is usually followed by "but" and rarely means the listener is curious.
9. Any given swearing: This generally indicates that emotions have gotten too hot to mentalize.

In MBT training, the television show *Columbo* is often used to discuss being curious but, in actuality, Columbo's "curiosity" is really a front for his already knowing the suspect is guilty and then cleverly tricking them into revealing their crimes, using many of the above MBT "swear words." That Columbo understands the motivations and mechanics of the crime and the culprit is not in doubt, but it is in reality not curiosity—it is what one would call a "misuse" of mentalizing. Indeed, even small children can recognize this conversational approach and will generally resent the maneuver. Perhaps a better example of genuine curiosity might be the cartoon character Curious George. His pleasant and earnest desire to learn is disarming and is more in line with the true curiosity we are striving for in the stance. Truly "not knowing," and with empathic feeling asking a person to "help me understand," are the goals of curiosity in the stance. As you work to understand, you are modeling the marked contingent mirroring discussed in Chap. 1. Many times, behaviorally, the meaning is conveyed in the body language (a slight head tilt, more direct eye contact, subtle shifts in body positioning) and verbal tone. Sometimes it is easier to consider examples in which people may say words that sound curious but their body language and tone of voice are conveying the exact opposite. For that reason, Columbo remains a good example as we discuss the concept of maintaining curiosity. So we ask you, dear reader, to consider using the phrases listed below to engage in curiosity that is essential for this leg of the mentalizing stance (Table 2.1).

In conclusion, these phrases will only "work their MBT magic" if you are ACTUALLY curious. If you are "putting on" curiosity like Columbo, especially with adolescents, it will come off as insincere. This in turn will activate epistemic

Table 2.1 Phrases that facilitate the "not knowing" stance

Hang on a minute, can we go back?
How did that come about?
What was the experience like?
How were you feeling in the moment (or in this moment)?
What do you make of what was said/was done/happened?
What about [the event] got you feeling that way?
Does it seem like I'm getting it?
Can you help me understand?

mistrust, *as it should.* Humans don't trust someone "being fake"—and this colloquial "BS detector" is how we evolved to avoid dangerous misuse of mentalizing by others. You really have to embrace what you do not know to have a "not knowing" stance!

Holding the Balance

As we said earlier, the stance is about active balance—and the concept of "holding the balance" is how an MBT therapist takes the mentalizing temperature of the session. One concept is to consider mentalizing as a light on a dimmer switch; indeed, you can concretely emphasize this with quick graphics on a page or whiteboard. Active explicit mentalizing requires a "balance" between the following four dimensions, as shown in Fig. 2.2.

Therefore, in a session, a therapist is observing how far along the above lines the therapist and patient are. Has the balance completely shifted to an extreme where there is an intense affect or absolute certainty about the other (i.e., psychic equivalence)? Is the patient completely in the modality of thoughts with little to no affect about themselves (i.e., in pretend mode)? Or is the patient perhaps displaying an intense affect with an excessive focus on getting you to "prove it" with action (i.e., in teleological mode)?

As the therapist considers the balance of the moment, the therapist is identifying whether or not mentalizing is occurring. Based on where the therapist might guess they are, the next step may be to shift one or more of these polarities to reactivate explicit mentalizing. The patient [and the therapist] must be able to shift their flexibility among these polarities to connect in a way that builds trust. This ongoing review of the balance will then prompt the therapist to either disengage from non-mentalizing, which is the third aspect of the stance, or highlight and promote the continuation of explicit mentalizing, which is the fourth aspect of the stance. Practically, the polarities can come to the rescue when non-mentalizing is "what's happening" by leaning hard toward the other pole—for example, saying "Well, what do you imagine I make of what you did?" to a patient fixated on their own experience.

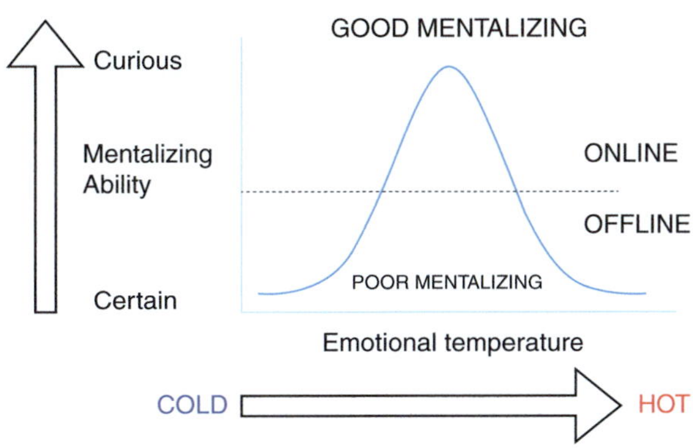

Fig. 2.2 The mentalizing bell curve

Disengaging from Non-mentalizing

Disengaging from non-mentalizing is crucial, because non-mentalizing begets non-mentalizing. Simply observing your patient, the family, or group continue along the path of non-mentalizing fosters mistrust, which will inhibit your attempts to grow mentalizing. Are your sessions a safe place whereby the patient "trusts," or are they seen as extensions of the mistrust (frequently in the family) that prompted therapy being sought? This disengagement from non-mentalizing is often "marked" by the therapist raising a hand in a plea to stop. Another playful way to encourage patients, families, or groups to stop non-mentalizing themselves is to create literal "pause buttons" out of play materials, to be pushed by anyone in the room to alert everyone to slow down a non-mentalizing moment. In the final maneuver introduced in this chapter, we find this is an opportunity for someone to "name" the moment as an example of a frequent pattern of non-mentalizing that the MBT team has co-constructed (the mentalizing loop: notice and name). Again, how a therapist might stop non-mentalizing will depend in part on recognizing which mentalizing failure is occurring and the general style you as a therapist have in bringing up challenging topics. There is no one "right way" to stop non-mentalizing. Creativity is encouraged. One example fondly remembered by an MBT therapist was his decision to get up and abruptly leave the room while the family was shouting. While out in the hall, the therapist was internally berating himself for such a clumsy move and actively wondering how the family was thinking of him. However, upon his return he found a more focused and quieter group recognizing that they had "scared the therapist." This reduction in the expressed affect—what we might term the *emotional temperature* in MBT—allowed both the therapist and the family members to "rewind" the recent event [the therapist leaving the room] through a mentalizing lens. In this instance, the therapist leaving worked in re-establishing mentalizing; however, a different therapist recalled such a move not working when tried in another session. An MBT therapist keeps their eye on mentalizing and if one approach is not successful, the therapist shifts the balance and re-engages in a different manner. There are few failures for an MBT therapist; rather, there are frequent opportunities to get curious—"Well, that didn't seem to work at all! What do you make of that?"—or it might be an opportunity to shift to a different polarity: "What could I have been thinking to try something so outrageous?"

Highlighting and Promoting Mentalizing

The final aspect of the four-legged stance (Fig. 2.2) is for the therapist to highlight and promote explicit mentalizing in the patient and themselves. Indeed, as we discussed in Chap. 1, learning from an attachment figure through modeling is key. Going back to the infant and parent, the child begins to learn their own mind through the mind of the other. This is done in that marked manner in order to promote further mentalizing. *The goal of mentalizing therapy is—to mentalize. That is it. Your earnest authors are not kidding. This is fundamental and foundational.* Emotions cannot be soothed and solutions cannot be discovered without this process. In the end, your goal in mentalizing therapy is to help the patient (or family or group) mentalize—and turn on explicit mentalizing when it goes "offline"—for themselves, thereby making the therapist obsolete. *The patient may need to learn additional skills, but our premise is that engendering active mentalizing is what allows the person to accept and in fact learn for themselves new approaches to the issues that brought them into therapy*. It is almost a magic trick: once mentalizing is back "online," one can consider other options and solutions, which, once unimaginable, come effortlessly to mind. For chronically suicidal youth, whose minds become frozen on teleological solutions like ending their own life, the ability to see that anything else is an option is literally a life-saving medicine. Figure 2.2 is often drawn in sessions to highlight for the patient the goal of MBT, which, as stated above, is to get mentalizing back online. This figure represents the concept that what we are aiming for in each session (and in daily life) is the ability to approach an issue with a curious state of mind where we will feel some emotional investment and have a sense of trust in discussing this difficult topic. We highlight that the MBT "sweet spot" is different for different people and even different for those people based on the topic and the other people involved in the situation or topic. So, actively modeling being curious, holding the balance, stopping non-mentalizing, and reinforcing and highlighting good mentalizing are skills we can learn and/or strengthen with the assistance of the therapist. If the therapist is successful in modeling and teaching patients to be more active in mentalizing, the patient can then recognize for themselves when they go offline and then can start to develop a road map for how to re-engage their own and others' mentalizing abilities. The next part of this chapter moves into the recognition of non-mentalizing modes and how to approach them such that the mentalizing sweet spot can be regained or obtained.

Mentalizing you, dear reader, we are imagining that by this point in the chapter, you are considering how you currently "do therapy." In fact, there are some readers who will likely believe "Hey, I already do this; why did I spend money on this book anyway?" Others may think "Hey, maybe there is something to this whole mentalizing thing, but how do I actually do it?"

Luckily, our response to both imagined reader reactions is "Fantastic! Tell me more about that! I am curious to know what similarities you see between MBT and your current approach." We might even say "Tell me where you are getting lost in what to do in sessions." Mentalizing: it even makes writing about mentalizing a bit easier (Fig. 2.3).

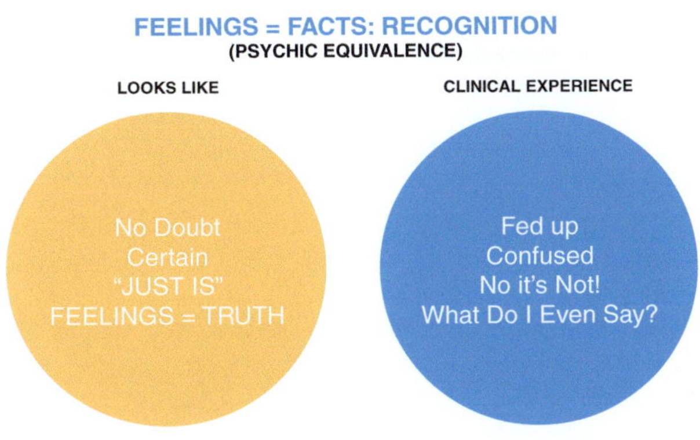

Fig. 2.3 Psychic equivalence: feelings = facts

Psychic Equivalence

We consider the next steps key to addressing non-mentalizing while in a session. Let us start with the two "emotionally hottest" non-mentalizing modes: the psychic equivalence and teleological modes. In both of these non-mentalizing modes, an intense affect rules the moment. For the therapist, these modes of thinking will usually very explicitly "knock you off the mentalizing stance," due to their intensity. As you respond in kind with non-mentalizing, the danger here is for the affect to blossom further, leading to a coercive cycle. Consider in life how after an intense argument ends you are often left wondering "How the [blank] did I [we] get here?" Both of these modes strongly pull the therapist to ACT. But be wary: these actions are not likely to lead to balanced explicit mentalizing for the patient or for you.

How might a therapist recognize psychic equivalence for the patient and themselves? First look for the intense affect that is generally followed by a sense of absolute certainty from the patient that the issue at hand "just is." Remember that for MBT, "just" is a four-letter word. Be watchful for the actual word or conversations that appear to lack any doubt. "I just needed to die, because Jessie dumping me meant my life was over," sobs Rebecca. "He's like his father—so lazy— he doesn't care about anyone but himself," remarks John's mother.

These absolute statements on a basic level scream "untruth!" Indeed, a common cognitive approach would be to ask the patient to consider the alternatives. The therapist should be wary about entering into a cognitive fact-finding mission at this time point in the session. That approach will most certainly only lead to further certainty and frustration for both parties. As the patient gets more certain—and certainly is starting to also be angry with you—the therapist is likely to be confused and fed up. Resist the temptation to argue. The patient is not ready to hear it. Remember we want to activate the attachment system and get on the epistemic trust superhighway; cognition is a dead end at this moment in time when the emotional temperature is too high. Mentalizing explicitly requires a balance between emotion and cognition and in this situation, you need to attend to the emotion (Fig. 2.4).

OK, if you cannot use logic, what should you do when faced with psychic equivalence? Instead, VALIDATE how they feel. Yes, validate. In fact, validate more than you have ever validated in your life. Validate until it feels weird. Probably then

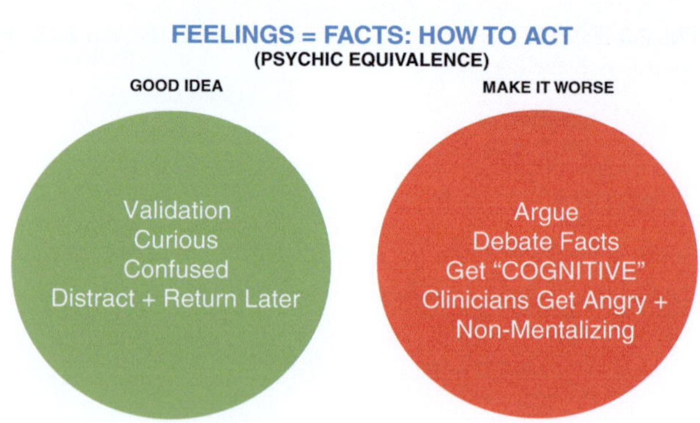

Fig. 2.4 Psychic equivalence: how to act

Fig. 2.5 Teleological mode: "prove-it" thinking. *w/o* without

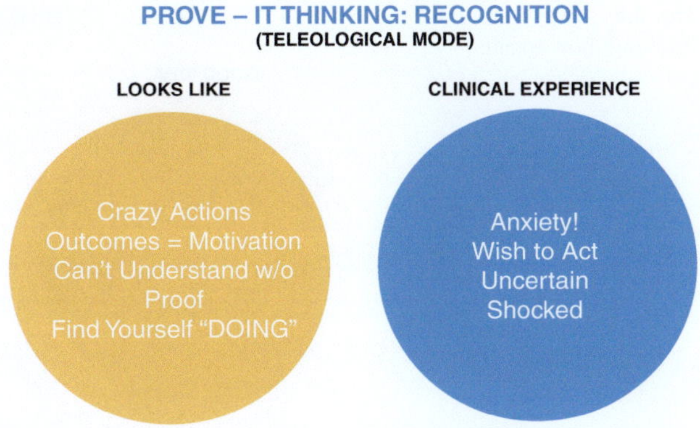

you might need to validate slightly more. Once you are done validating, do it again. Then pivot to the next feeling you are actually having [see above]—yep, confusion. Here's your chance to use the mentalizing stance [yeah!]—model the "not knowing" stance. Wonder together about this curious moment in time. If after validating and modeling curiosity, the affect and certainty remain too elevated, agree to move on (distract) to a different topic for now and see if using the balance leg of the stance can provide a different perspective. [Remember the polarities.] Again, the goal is to return to a balanced mentalizing stance. If/when you and the patient can achieve this flexible stance, then try cognitive reframing or any other skills or techniques to problem solve. Consider the proverb "Don't spit into the wind." An MBT therapist knows to validate and then save the skills until after the wind [affect] has died down. A beautiful moment of validation occurs in the Pixar movie *Inside Out*. In a pivotal scene, Joy is relentlessly trying to make another character [just] be happy and move on. The character only devolves further into tears and inaction. Here Sadness steps in to validate how bad the character feels. They spend a few moments where the other character feels held by sadness. With that validation, the character is able to reorganize and move through their sadness, allowing them to move forward (Fig. 2.5).

Teleological Mode

The next affectively hot mode of thinking is teleological. In this mode, the patient is threatening to act in certain extreme ways or is pleading with you, the therapist, to act. In this way, the intensity of the task prompts a large amount of anxiety in the therapist. A therapist will find themselves blurring a boundary that is normally firmly held or using an action to "prove" how serious and concerned the therapist is in response to the patient's needs. Five more minutes every session, excessive communication between sessions, refilling of medication, adding new medications, or treatments without sound reasons are but a few examples. Like most anxiety, the more you give in to the anxiety, the more the patient needs you to keep "proving" you care. If the only way for a person to "prove concern" is to "do something," eventually that relationship will break on a fault line. In this way, we discuss the

Fig. 2.6 "Prove-it" thinking: how to act

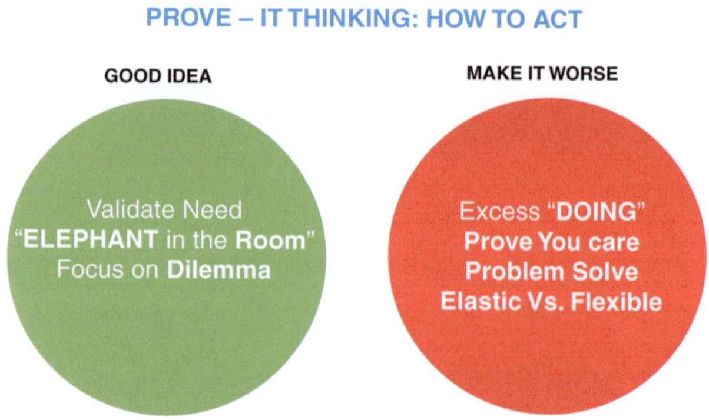

Fig. 2.7 Pretend mode

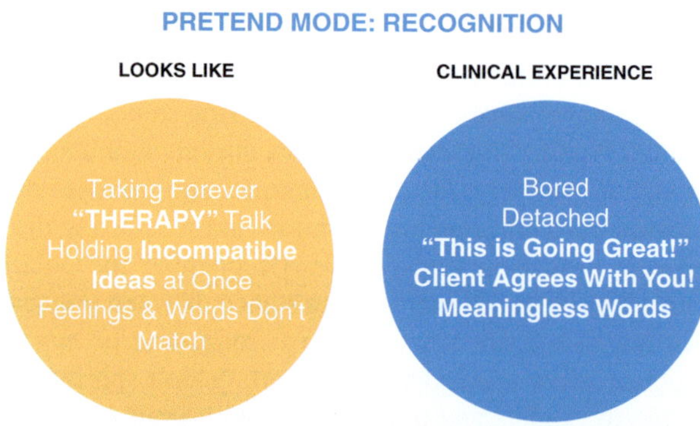

difference between a therapist (and patient) being flexible versus elastic. Flexible is a preferred aspect of mentalizing—but teleological mode actually pulls you to become elastic. The problem with elastic is that it either breaks or snaps back. Suddenly outwardly annoyed at all the "extra" ways in which they have been providing care, the therapist puts the brakes on and the wheels come off (Fig. 2.6).

So how do you move the therapy out of teleological processes? As in psychic equivalence, you must FIRST validate the patient's experience. Again, this is a marked contingent mirroring of the patient that is not meant to agree or join with the validation, especially when the patient might be discussing suicide, self-harm, or deep pain or rage. But it is validation—giving the patient a sense that you are with them as they feel these emotions. It would do no one any good, however, if you and the patient continued to stay here, so next, the therapist needs to acknowledge the "elephant in the room." The hope is that by verbalizing the problem, the therapist can share the dilemma with the patient and join together in creating a path forward. "I hear you, Robin; you are so, so sad and hurt that you FEEL like dying. I can see it in your face and in the way you're sitting. I hear that you want me to prescribe more sleep medications BECAUSE the pain feels like more than you can bear. But that medication really won't help. I do want to help—I do—but we need to talk more and see about a different plan that doesn't include that medication. Can we do that? But first I want to hear more about how the rest of the day went. Can we start after you got his message breaking up with you?" (Fig. 2.7).

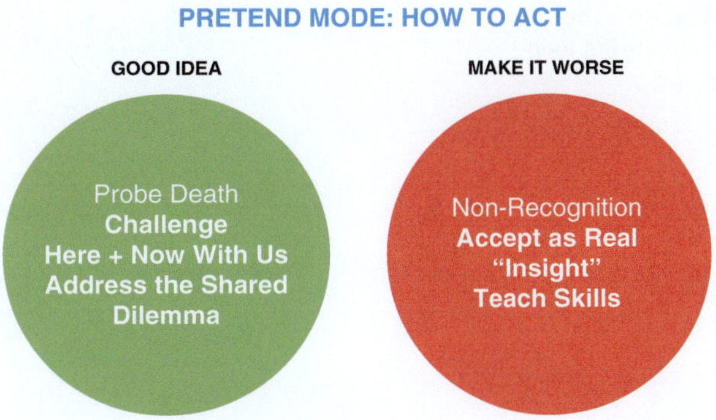

Fig. 2.8 Pretend mode: how to act

Pretend Mode

On the surface, pretend mode doesn't feel as intensely uncomfortable as the first two modes. However, pretend mode is equally problematic, in that months and years might go by without any significant progress made in treatment. In pretend mode, both the patient and therapist can fall into pretending the treatment is working. Somehow the patient never seems to use those insights or skills learned in sessions, but they can speak eloquently about how much treatment is helping them—even if they remain depressed, use substances, fall into the same relationship traps, and have suicidal thoughts or are prone to self-injurious acts. Indeed, in this mode the problem often is LACK OF AFFECT. For whatever reason, the patient is not accessing their emotions and the sessions will have a dreamy or hazy air to them. Therapists will often feel a great deal of boredom (and then guilt for thinking this) or will be detached and distracted in a session. Creating your grocery list while the patient discusses their insights about their mother should be a big WAKE-UP call for the therapist that pretend mode is firmly engaged. Pretend mode in many ways is "easy." The therapist and the patient have a sense that treatment is working and a strong desire to not really discuss how the patient can't stop drinking because that would "just" be too much effort. They wouldn't want to rock the boat after all (Fig. 2.8).

The key to taking on pretend mode is to rock the boat. Turn up the affective temperature. Bring the dilemma right into the here and now of the session. A therapist might remark that they are lost or feeling distracted in the session. They can invite the patient to join in on considering why that might be, or they can issue a challenge by probing the depth. "Sarah, I might be off base here, but I am wondering what you REALLY think about deep breathing. I wonder if you actually think it is a load of crap. I say this because just now we were talking about how you were having a horrible panic attack but didn't bring up using these skills we've practiced several times. You have told me it's good, but I'm not so sure. What do you think? Am I off base?"

Is challenge or probing the depth just picking a fight? When do you know if you should probe or accept that the patient is feeling "good" when you check in? Again, we focus you back on the affective tone of the room as well as the context of the

Fig. 2.9 The mentalizing loop

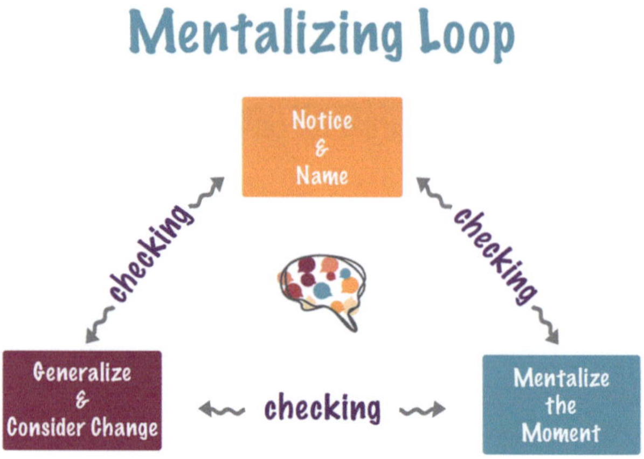

conversation. Yes the patient might really be good—if you can see how connected their actions, thoughts, and feelings are to the topics at hand. Nevertheless, if there appears to be a disconnect and you have your inner Spidey sense tingling with boredom, pretend mode should be considered turned on. It is up to you, the therapist, to engage the elephant in the room (Fig. 2.9).

Notice and Name: The Mentalizing Loop

Hopefully, by this point, mentalizing is starting to make a bit of sense. You can see how the stance is designed to activate epistemic trust and help you recognize mentalizing or the lack thereof. You are starting to see how the three non-mentalizing modes can interrupt progress in treatment and maybe have a few ideas about how to re-engage in flexible explicit mentalizing. Nevertheless, how does this really connect to therapy sessions?

Remember how we discussed turning mentalizing on and off? In fact, every person has certain triggers that turn mentalizing off, as we noted in Chap. 1, since no one is perfectly mentalized by their caregivers. That weird term *alien self*—we're bringing it back up again. It is important! Well patients likely have those areas involved in their reasons for coming to therapy. So you, as the therapist, are dutifully staying on task by turning mentalizing up or on when it comes to those specific topics. As you do this, patterns will emerge that are visible to you and the patient. This is not insight, per se, but more a procedural blind-spot discovery that the patient needs help mentalizing. In MBT therapy, we call this concept *notice and name*. It is through this iterative process (see Fig. 2.9) that this non-mentalized blind spot is brought out into the light to examine and consider its relevance to the identified problem(s) that brought the patient into treatment. If the patient, family, and you agree there is relevance, then the goal is to name the process. Why name it? Well, simply put, naming something gives everyone access to that "something." In naming it, you allow the patient to keep some continuity between sessions about these non-mentalized blind spots. As in any treatment, forward progress can come in fits and starts. Having a shorthand way to "pause" the action when the pattern re-emerges can help keep the focus on moving treatment forward.

Conclusion

This chapter has hopefully introduced you to the techniques that are foundational to a mentalizing treatment approach. In review, these are the four legs of the mentalizing stance, the identification of and approaches to the three non-mentalizing modes of action, and the development of session continuity by utilization of the mentalizing loop (notice and name). We encourage you to review the videos that accompany this chapter and refer back to them when you are considering how to approach treatment in a mentalizing manner.

Acknowledgments The author would like to acknowledge Anna Freud Centre for Children and Families and their team in their efforts towards educating clinicians in mentalization-based theory and practice. The following link describes the progression of training in the general MBT model. A similar pathway exists for working with adolescents, children, youth, and families. https://www.annafreud.org/training/mentalization-based-treatment-training/mbt-training-programme/

Suggested Reading

1. Anna Freud National Centre for Children and Families. Mentalization-based treatment for adolescence (MBT-A) training programme. https://www.annafreud.org/training/mentalization-based-treatment-training/mbt-a-training-programme/. Accessed 1 Dec 2019.

Mentalizing in Family Work

3

Chris W. Grimes and Owen Muir

Introduction

For many therapists, family work can feel overwhelming. It has been our experience that for many youth in the USA, at least, the focus is generally on individual treatment. A common theme from our work with parents is that their experience of therapy leaves them in the dark. They bring the young person to the session, wait outside, and, in far too many cases, do not have regular conversations or sessions with the young person and the therapist in the room. This is puzzling for a mentalizing therapist. How can the work be isolated from individuals who are helping shape the young person, struggle with the young person, and ultimately need to be engaged in the long-term development of new strategies so as to make the therapist obsolete?

However, if we take our initial words—"feel overwhelming"—it can start to make a bit of sense; trying to hold one person's mind in mind is one thing, but a room full of people? That's a nice way to turn off mentalizing, when you think about it! From a mentalizing perspective, family therapy should not, as the kids say, "suck." While the adults may not use that word, they too can find family therapy to be uncomfortable, as often their experience of doing family work can feel like they are being "blamed," and shame is a powerful inhibitor of the mentalizing mind.

This, dear reader, is where we say, "Bring on the mentalizing!" As a therapist, your biggest impact will be in assisting not just the young person but also their mentalizing team. You have to make the entire team into a mentalizing powerhouse, and that doesn't necessarily happen by working only with the individual. How do we learn our minds? By first seeing them mirrored in those who care for us [1].

C. W. Grimes (✉)
Menninger Department of Psychiatry and Behavioral Sciences, Baylor College of Medicine, Houston, TX, USA

O. Muir
Brooklyn Minds Psychiatry, Brooklyn, NY, USA

L. L. Williams, O. Muir (eds.), *Adolescent Suicide and Self-Injury*,
https://doi.org/10.1007/978-3-030-42875-4_3

Family therapy can be a space to learn better ways to respond to self-harm for both the young person and their parents. As we said earlier, it is a common (almost universal) experience that parents caring for young people who are suicidal or engage in self-injury feel enormous shame, which many times is masked by anger and increasingly contentious behavioral controls designed to keep the young person safe. Therapy needs to hold their minds in mind as well and help promote their competence just as much as we work to help the young person. Honor that the room is full of anxious people, including yourself, but take a steady breath, get your balance, and mentalize.

This chapter will discuss the following:

1. Initial family mentalizing assessment and formulation
2. Promoting the mentalizing stance within the family
   (a) Holding the balance
   (b) Highlighting good mentalizing
   (c) Disengaging from non-mentalizing
3. The mentalizing loop, with examples

In order to assist you, dear reader, in learning these objectives, the chapter will review one case to highlight the important aspects of using mentalizing in family work.

Case Introduction

I find that when I meet a young person and family, it's best to listen, stay in the moment, and show genuine interest and curiosity about each member and the family system as a whole. What does the family have to tell me? What do they misunderstand about one another? Do the members find each other confusing at times? In my curiosity, I encourage the family members to be their own experts as they share their experiences. I slow them down so we can together think about their minds in the moment, as they share. I ask, "What's it's like to talk about this right now with me or your family member? Do others know you feel this way?" I check out if others have understood their story as they are telling it in the moment. Are they learning something new about one another as they begin to allow me to know them? I help them imagine together about what they each would like to learn about themselves and others in the family process. I reflect openly on the astonishing ability they have to articulate how they feel; sit with them during times when they express uncertainty, suicidality, helplessness, and shame; and imagine with them what they want to be different.

Lydia is a 12-year-old, who has struggled throughout her entire life with maintaining relationships, first with family members and now increasingly at school. Her parents describe Lydia as "needy," "demanding," "clingy," and "manipulative," and say that friends tire of her endless "narcissism" and intensity.

Lydia's Mom, Linda, loves her children but feels overwhelmed and exhausted, and finds herself in verbal and physical battles with Lydia. Her father, Larry, works long hours, leaving her mother as the primary caregiver of Lydia and her young brother. From Linda's perspective, Lydia demands attention and is competitive for her father's affection. She believes that Lydia turns into a different kid when her father is around. In moments of conflict, Mom acknowledges that she thinks Lydia sees her as "dumb," which leads her to get defensive, followed by giving Lydia a consequence (usually taking her phone away). While Lydia doesn't say these words usually, Mom is *certain* that Lydia thinks this about her. Mom often feels misunderstood and alone with the kids, especially when Dad is away. She desperately wants a parenting partner and is unhappy in her marriage. She responds with intense reactions to Lydia, almost as though she herself is another teen. She has started to give in to Lydia's demands to avoid long nights of battle with her, which often end with Lydia cutting herself.

Larry, Lydia's father, acknowledges he is apart from his family much of the time. He is *clear* that Lydia is "nuts" and wonders why she has to make things so difficult for herself and her family. He has a view of how Lydia "should" be and operates according to this view. He sees any behavior that is not in accordance with his view of how a family should work as "bad." Larry indicates that when he returns home, Lydia is "in his face," demanding attention. Dad *knows* that Lydia makes things up, has little empathy, and cares little about how her behavior impacts the family. He sees her self-injury as manipulation and downplays her suicidality, indicating that she learned this from a friend, from school, or through the media. He indicates that Mom lets Lydia walk all over her. His solution is that Lydia *just* needs to focus more on school and behave. When her father returns from being away on a business trip, Lydia's aggression seems to intensify with her mother until Dad takes over in powerful, rejecting, and at times *physical* ways. Both parents believe the self-injury is a way for her to seek attention after she does something wrong. Here's a question for you, dear reader: What modes of non-mentalizing do we see in these statements?

From Lydia's perspective, she doesn't think her mother is dumb, but she *really believes* that her mother doesn't like her very much. She worries that her mother is not happy and *believes* that she takes her stress out on her. She wonders why when her Dad comes home, her Mom seems to turn meaner. She is scared at times of her father's temper but explains that he has a right to be so angry. Lydia describes herself as an "idiot," "lonely," and without any friends. Lydia *insists* that her family doesn't care about her, and she fantasizes about being in another family. After her rages, she feels extreme guilt and cuts herself. After cutting, the pain subsides and she does everything she can to get back in good graces with her mother. She was bullied early on in second grade and had to repeat that grade, and this was, followed by a move to another school. This rejection by others has become evidence to Lydia that she is unlovable, stupid, alone, and a burden. She knows she is a bad sister and daughter, and that the rest of her family would be better without her (see Box 3.1).

Box 3.1

As your writer, I will confess that early experiences of "patients" involving managed care, poverty, trauma, and severe mental illness led me to "burn out." This "in-the-trench" work left me feeling powerless, overwhelmed, and questioning how to bring about change. I needed a life raft but didn't know that mentalizing is what I needed as a new clinician. This is particularly true of family systems experiencing chronic suicidality and self-injury. Questions abound: Where do you even begin? What if I say the wrong thing? I can't deal with blood very well. What if a patient dies? What did graduate school say about this? Can I stop a kid from cutting himself or herself? What do I do if the session makes things worse? Learning and applying mentalizing therapy has given me a toolbox that fixes not just my life raft but also those of the families I work with. I am always reminded of a flight attendant's safety briefing, in which parents are asked to put on their own oxygen masks first. This is a great way to consider mentalizing therapy: it needs to happen with the adults and then the young people. That is what keeps us all safe.

Initial Family Mentalizing Assessment and Formulation

We recognize that there are "facts" you need to gather as you meet a new patient/family. If you are practicing the mentalizing stance while working, there should hopefully be much to glean from the fact-finding beginnings; indeed, in Chap. 4 we will discuss a mentalizing activity you can utilize right at the start to get the mentalizing juices flowing.

So, as we review the above information, what stands out to you as it relates to mentalizing abilities? This is an important exercise to consider how well each person mentalizes, as this will help you develop an assessment that goes beyond *Diagnostic and Statistical Manual of Mental Disorders, Fifth Edition* (DSM-5) diagnoses and is hopefully more dimensional and representative of the core concerns that bring the young person and family to your office. We recognize that family work may happen in a variety of ways; you may be tasked with doing both individual and family work, or perhaps you are part of a larger team that allows you to focus on the family. Each approach has unique benefits and challenges that are beyond the scope of this chapter; however, we urge you to consider how to keep mentalizing going regardless of the system challenges. Family therapy does not always need to include every family member in every session. At times, issues may arise where it makes more sense to have a separate session to allow for improved mentalization. So, as you consider your structure with a family, we want you to remember to be FLEXIBLE but not elastic—a key component of successful mentalizing.

An important concept to clarify here is that in mentalizing therapy we consider the formulation as a verb, not a noun. By this we mean that the formulation should change based on updated experiences and observations. An assessment and formulation should be co-constructed with the family so there is a shared purpose to the treatment. A mentor, Efrain Bleiberg, MD, is fond of saying we can all "own 2% of the problem." By suggesting this idea early on (and modeling this where you can we can, as therapists), we hope to instill a sense of agency, willingness, inquisitiveness, and openness throughout the assessment process.

Example Formulation

Lydia is a young girl who is struggling with her sense of isolation, fear, and disgust, and she is certain that she is bad and worthy of being punished. Each parent themselves appears to have very certain thoughts about why Lydia feels and acts in these ways; however, their own emotions are rarely discussed beyond anger. It appears that as negative feelings are not readily expressed or understood, the family members find themselves in coercive and contentious verbal and physical arguments, leaving both sides exhausted and giving way to a sense of incompetence and hopelessness. Lydia sees her self-injury as an expression of these ugly emotions, providing initial evidence of the *alien self* and a sense of relief that quickly morphs into a growing sense of hopelessness and incompetence that both Lydia and her family feel. The parents appear to have challenges within their relationship that are not yet fully understood. The therapist will want to support the parents' development of a more cohesive mentalizing parenting team, by which we mean each parent mentalizing themselves and their partner in addition to Lydia and her brother.

Overall, there are a great number of mentalizing challenges exhibited by each family member; each mode of mentalizing failures could be found in the assessment process. We consider Fig. 3.1 a helpful tool to explain to a family the pattern that frequently emerges when young people and their families are struggling with serious mental health challenges.

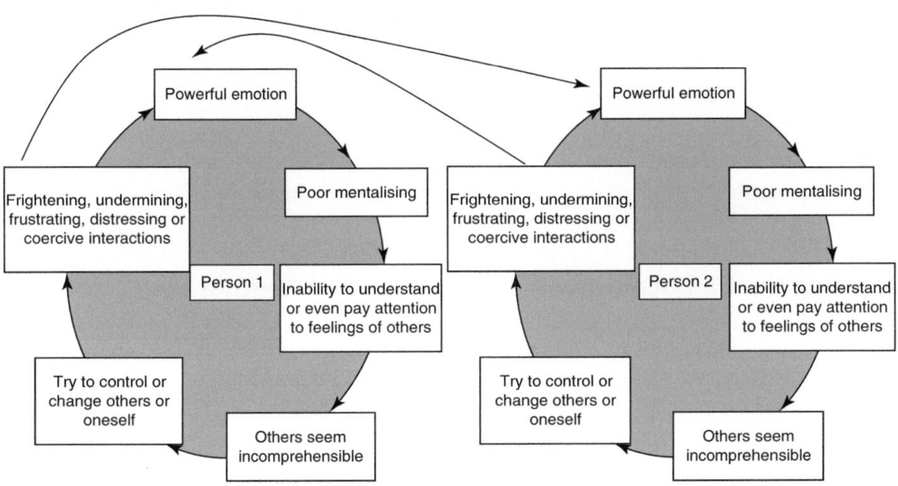

Fig. 3.1 Vicious cycles of non-mentalizing in families

Promoting the Mentalizing Stance in Therapy

Holding the Balance: Curiosity

As we mentalize, we really want to get to know the family and, initially, what it's like to be in that family. Lydia struggles though to reach out for support, so staying curious with her and being willing to be with her in the moment can be as powerful as anything. After the initial assessment and the development of the formulation, the therapist presents these ideas to the family and considers what they may have gotten "right" and also, just as importantly, what the therapist may have gotten "wrong" or missed about the challenges the family faces.

In being curious about the family/individual stories, we support the family in building a sense of identity, illuminating values, and identifying strengths, while questioning long-held and possibly rigid beliefs and automatic responses. We allow them the space to find the words to describe who they are and what they want. I find that clients appreciate the interest and attention I give to their stories. Before I know it, I have learned so much about them and feel more about what it's like to be them in their family. We do inquire and, in doing so, support the mentalizing process. We want the client to be curious about their experience and the experience of others in their family. How does Dad's mind work? Why does Lydia work so desperately to convince me to give her more time on her phone? What would my children be like if I were Linda? Could I imagine feeling like killing myself if I were her?

I wonder aloud with the entire family about how each member might feel when the father is at home away from work. How does it feel if you are Mom, Dad, or Lydia? Being curious about anything in a session can support mentalizing. I get confused and share my confusion openly with Dad when he says something about Lydia that doesn't fit with how I see him. During my work with the family, I strive to stay curious, validate perspectives, and then help them generate other ideas rather than telling them my perspective. However, at times I may suggest openly "I wonder…" and gently challenge the father to bring mentalizing back online. With Mom, Lydia is convinced that Mom doesn't love her. In sessions, we reflect on what else might be in her Mom's mind. I don't dismiss what is in her mind, only encourage her to stay curious when she feels she "knows" something about her mother.

Holding the Balance: Slowing Down/Emotion Regulation

I can easily get swept away when families tell their story, especially their side of the story. The American modern family system is full of colorful dynamics to explore, and some members will be sure you understand their perspective before you can even imagine what is going on in someone else's mind. By slowing things down, we support mentalizing.

Help the parents and adolescents think about how to strengthen their own emotion regulation through the development of "pause buttons" and by modeling slowing down in sessions to develop explicit mentalizing. While we don't have to move at a snail's pace, it is important that everyone has an opportunity to feel heard and supported. The slowing down allows time for the mentalizing to get back online, to avoid misunderstandings in the first place.

I imagine that everyone in a family wants to be heard and understood, and would like things to be different. The idea that a family might get to a place where they can slow themselves down, look at themselves, and say, "Hey, let's try something different" is the ultimate milestone for families to achieve. The family develops a sort of combined agency that allows them to identify when they are moving too quickly, fighting for control. We work to slow down, rewind even, and then encourage the family to appreciate what it is actually like to slow down. Can they imagine doing this themselves?

In Lydia's family, a common pattern the therapist begins to notice is that everyone wants to be in control of the conversation. As things slow down, the family members learn more about the *why*. Each person is able to reflect on feeling unheard and helpless when they don't feel understood. Together, the family reflects on more about how each person may look from the outside when they are feeling misunderstood. This allows the family to look at themselves from the outside and use feedback from the therapist and—most importantly—from one another to identify non-mentalizing and appreciate what it feels like for everyone, including themselves, in the moment.

Holding the Balance: The Affect Focus

When working with this family, I often wonder what is beneath the anxiety, coercion, explosiveness, and name-calling. Lydia is often described as a drama queen, too sensitive and demanding, oppositional defiant, and unemotional. I quickly find myself sick of the labels and wonder more about what it feels like for everyone to be in this family system. With gentle curiosity, I inquire about her affect and what might be going on in Lydia's mind when her parents call her "dramatic." How does she feel and what does she think about herself when she hears this? Maybe in the moments when others experience her as "dramatic," she feels quite desperate, lonely, and overwhelmed, and desires to be anyone but herself. As a family, it might be worth acknowledging that these feelings exist and that how we think about one another matters. When emotions are identified, be willing to slow down and even allow for a bit of silence to sit with them. Often, the mentalizing therapist will suggest, "Can we just sit with this for a moment? I really am trying to get a sense of what it feels like for each of you as we sit together right now."

As treatment progresses, the therapist notices that her parents tended to respond to Lydia's distress in a variety of ways: "Lydia, you are too sensitive," "Lydia, you are not making any sense." Support them in thinking together about what might be going on for Lydia. What does it mean to be sensitive? I wonder why what she is saying is not making any sense. "Lydia, do you know what your parents mean by too demanding?" Helping parents and kids use feeling words and really think about how these feelings show up in the family is a helpful way to orient yourself in sessions. We might imagine someone feels a certain way but, at the same time, we could get it wrong. Encourage the family to "check out" with others if they are getting it right. Emotions allow us to better understand why we do what we do. Sharing emotions in moments when others are really interested and vulnerable supports the healing process.

Holding the Balance: The "Here and Now" Focus

Orienting your sessions to the "here and now" activates the attachment system in therapeutic relationships. When we are talking about what is happening in the room, we are exploring the moment and learning from the moment. This turns up the emotional temperature, knocking families out of pretend mode. For instance, we must be sensitive to the idea of not aligning with one member or the other. It's also important to call out this "elephant in the room" if you are sensing that others might be feeling that you are taking sides. This demonstrates curiosity around similar dynamics that might be happening within the family. Similarly to how Irvin Yalom, PhD, discusses "process illumination" in group work [2], the mentalizing therapist works to illuminate moments of mentalizing in the moment within family sessions.

Holding the Balance: Perspective-Taking

Understanding what it's like to be a family member is important. The clinician should imagine what it's like for the parent not just outside a session but also inside a session. What is it like for their children to sit with parents in these sessions with a new person hearing their struggles? Often I hear parents say, "I should know what to do as a parent when my child is hurting." They also ask how much to openly discuss suicidality and self-injury with their kids. They wonder if they should search their bodies and rooms, or sleep in the same room with their child. Home is not a hospital; nor can a hospital become a child's home and magically keep them safe.

Mentalizing helps parents become curious about their child's behavior and provides a place for them to explore the mind of their child. I try to help families replace exclamation points with question marks at the ends of sentences. "Why is she isolating!" With mentalization-based treatment (MBT), this can become "*Why* is she isolating?" I then highlight the emotional difference between these sentences for families—for example, the difference between "He just wants attention!" and "Does he *want* attention?" Parents begin to understand what they bring to the table and actually speak about this to their kids as a way to model taking ownership without spiraling into shame. How do we support one another in a more effective manner to promote growth and competence?

Perspective-taking is a powerful tool for the therapist seeking to help the family explore new ways of seeing each other and the problems before them [3]. Slowing down, use of role play, and other activities like a "brain scan" (see Chap. 4) help the family consider others' points of view [4]. Appreciate how Lydia views herself in the context of her family and other relationships. How does she see things, and can I trust that she is sharing a genuine perspective? The more we can think about what others are thinking and feeling, and how they see the world, the less incomprehensible others become.

Help parents understand how their perspective of the world might be experienced by their child. How does their child see them, experience them? Lydia hasn't been sure she really is cared about, especially since her brother was born. Mom's ability to provide an adequate amount of mirroring given understandable circumstances reflects how Lydia may have experienced significant loneliness and pain related to her primary attachment figure. Why is it so important to Larry that he cannot listen to others' perspectives right now? Larry initially feels like an engima to the therapist and the family. How best to support Larry in order for him to discuss his perspective and how he feels is equally important for this family.

Highlighting Good or Improved Mentalizing: Humility

As a clinician, the more I do this work, the more I realize I really know very little. I have become one of the world's leading authorities in getting it wrong. The mentalizing stance provides me with security within this work. I know I very much rely on relationships to keep me afloat and to help me get back on track. It's not easy asking for help, especially if there is a risk involved. Letting the family know that I'm going to make mistakes and that I very much hope to own my mistakes models agency and humility. I'm careful not to mock myself or self-deprecate, but I'm open to hearing what it might be like during one of my goofs. I will often reference the support I get from others on my treatment team in helping me keep my mentalizing online in the face of my own mistakes making me feel small and ashamed.

Highlighting Good or Improved Mentalizing: Humor

Given that we work in the field of human suffering and as clinicians are exposed to this suffering, it is important to me to appreciate the moments with families where laughter can be had. These moments are like "attachment catnip," promoting secure attachments. In order to say "something funny," you have to comprehend the mind of the listener and often trip it up in some unexpected way. This makes humor inherently a mentalizing task. It might be a moment in the family discussion where they look at each other and burst into laughter or a joke. The idea that we might even be able to laugh at ourselves is nice mentalizing. We can look at ourselves from the outside and say, "Wow, in all this suffering I'm finding moments, and how powerful it is when I can share these with families." Often, humor gets in the way of real work as well, and we can wonder with the family what function it serves in those moments. Although Lydia and her family have had sincere moments of sitting with pain and uncertainty, they have also had intimate moments where they could step back and laugh or share a memory.

Highlighting Good or Improved Mentalizing: Impact Awareness

Understanding that any therapy may bring any unresolved family-of-origin issues and intergenerational traumas into the relationships is an important concept for recognizing impact awareness [4]. No relationship is more intense emotionally than those of our family [3]. Realizing this fact, these relationships can be the most loving *and* the most hurtful of all relationships. Family is the hardest to mentalize for most people! Appreciating how various systems and interpersonal factors impact the adolescent and family is crucial to really mentalize them. Helping the family to step back and consider all of this can be a powerful intervention. Sure, they can each own a small percentage of the problem—remember the 2% rule above—but a lot may be out of their control. Often, I will exaggerate this, in a manner similar to that of the marked, contingent mirroring discussed in Chap. 1.

Generating mentalizing within the family strengthens behavioral control if there is the willingness to really appreciate the impact we have on one another. There is a balance of shaming and supporting self-awareness. Impact awareness involves appreciating how we collide with one another and the resulting experiences. Help the parent slow down, consider other points of view, and reflect on what they may be inadvertently or unconsciously contributing to the distress of the adolescent. Typically, there is already enough self and other blame to go around, but helping them understand they do play a role and how to change on their part will impact the child. All of this takes a certain amount of risk on the part of the parents. If you push or hold boundaries, you will see your children respond in new ways, with new emotional experiences and strong emotions. Parents often feel they should "just" (there is that word again!) know and they wonder why their child is the one who is so self-destructive. They misinterpret their child's behavior because their mentalizing has gone offline. Remember that being scared turns off mentalizing, and what could be scarier than hearing that your child wants to die? If I have never been suicidal or depressed or struggling to find comfort and security in others, how can I really know? While a parent may not have experienced these feelings, they must want to know so that the child can feel safe to tell them.

Highlighting Good or Improved Mentalizing: Forgiveness

Ultimately, this is what we are moving toward. Mentalizing helps the family consider a rupture and move into a "more curious, less furious" way. It takes time to forgive but, by supporting the mentalizing interactions, the family members work through understanding how misunderstood they have each felt. With support, Lydia's parents are able to acknowledge to Lydia that they have not handled various situations in a very helpful way. Acknowledging that you haven't got it right, no matter who you are, allows for more flexibility that there really can be a "reset" or a "mentalizing do-over."

Support the family in examining ruptures (inside or outside the session) in a mentalizing fashion. Inverted roles (see Chap. 4) are helpful here because you can get them to imagine what it has been like from other family members' perspectives related to the rupture [3]. This was helpful when Lydia's mother found a bloody towel with a pencil sharper blade in Lydia's bathroom. "What was it like, Lydia, to learn that your Mom found this? What do you imagine she was thinking? What do you think she told Dad when he came home?" "How did Lydia feel when she realized you found out, Mom?" "How did we get here, Lydia? Can you help us understand?" How did the parents handle their responses then? What could have been done differently from everyone's perspective? One goal might be for the parents to pause themselves in the midst of finding Lydia self-harmed and do something different. It's really hard to be curious, and the mentalizing therapist encourages the family to think about what they might do differently, or specifically how the child would have preferred the parents to handle the situation.

Disengaging from Non-mentalizing: Psychic Equivalence

Particularly in the context of their relationship, and in moments of conflict, both Lydia and her mother can each become absolutely certain about what the other thinking and feeling (psychic equivalence). These moments usually accompany arguments, long and intense debates, anger, and more non-mentalizing. During a session, Lydia's mother suggests that maybe they need to reduce her screen time because she isolates so much from the rest of her family (psychic equivalence). Coercive move, mom! Mom is certain that social media time is more important than family time for Lydia. Mom's thinking in the moment suggests she "knows" that excessive social media is responsible for Lydia isolating from the family. Mom's parenting response is teleological in nature, as she indicates that maybe Lydia can "prove" to her mother that she does care about her family by having less time on her screens. Lydia snaps in a rage, shouting, "Bullshit! Why do you punish me for no reason!" To Lydia, this becomes evidence that her Mom "really doesn't love her," which increases her certainty about Mom. How could her Mom accuse her of not loving the family?! As we can see, non-mentalizing leads to more non-mentalizing very quickly, and no one is feeling very understood.

Slow the family down, using the mentalizing hand (gently raise your hands in the air as if stopping traffic) and share your mind with the family. "Can we take a pause here?" Let them know that you are feeling confused and want to make sure you understand everyone's perspective and how we got here. Model validation and support this process openly. Does anyone have any ideas? What is Lydia feeling right now? "Maybe we can think about Lydia's experience in the moment. Would that be OK, Lydia? I wonder how Mom comes to think that you don't want to spend time with your family. Maybe you can check that out. Why do you think Mom is punishing you? Lydia, what are other reasons why Mom might be doing what she is doing?"

Use the brain scan technique [3] described in Chap. 4 to support Mom and Lydia in considering what is actually in each other's minds and behind their behaviors. With support, Lydia discusses the experience she has of her mother when Mom is being "mean," what it looks like from her perspective, and what it feels like. The therapist asks, "Lydia, can we be curious with Mom as to why she responds this way when you isolate? Can you check in with her?" Lydia explains that she experiences her mother as disappointed in her and she wonders if her family would be better off without her. In these moments she is certain she is the problem in her family and the loneliness and emptiness overwhelm her. She finds relief in self-injury and isolates, and she is able to reflect on these moments with her Mom openly. She indicates that she doesn't share these moments with Mom because her parents become overly concerned, intrusive, and coercive. This is why her screen time is important to her because it helps her not feel so lonely and distracts her from her emotions. Mom indicates that she is willing to try something different in her response if Lydia can share more openly what is going on inside her. Lydia helps Mom understand how to approach her in these moments. Lydia is able to help Mom to learn more about how sensitive she is to Mom's verbal and non-verbal responses. She tearfully discusses how she assumes Mom's love for her is tenuous. The therapist supports the family in moving away from being certain, coercive, and reactive and toward being curious, collaborative, and willing to sit with uncertainty, especially in moments of helplessness and overwhelming emotions.

Disengaging from Non-mentalizing: Pretend Mode

During a session, the family begins discussing a recent self-injury episode, wondering aloud about how to respond to moments when they are unsure if Lydia is safe. Mom expresses struggling to know how to understand and respond to Lydia's self-injury and is interested in Lydia letting her into her world. Lydia makes it clear she has no intention of sharing with her. Dad goes on to lecture Lydia for the next few minutes about how important it is to live within the family values and says that if she doesn't start owning her behavior, she will have a hard time as an adult. Lydia shouts at her parents that they just need to leave her alone and let her do what she wants, as she "doesn't need them" (pretend mode). She indicates she might open up more if they stop their incessant punishments. Mom responds quickly by suggesting that maybe she needs to go to hospital if she isn't going to open up and be a part of the family. Lydia indicates that she "doesn't care" and it "doesn't really matter" that this makes her parents sad (pretend mode). She says that they don't give her any freedom, as evidenced by her parents taking her bedroom door off its hinges, Mom sleeping in the same room as her, and Dad and Mom locking up all the "sharps" in the house. These comments tend to increase the parents' anxiety about Lydia's safety, and they respond in more teleological ways that feel coercive and confusing (in efforts to keep her "safe").

When you have a sense of the pretend mode in the moment, don't get wrapped up in trying to understand the pretense. You can be empathic while not accepting what the person is saying as real. The therapist investigates more, digging deeper to fully appreciate what is happening in the moment. Stick with the stance and be curious… "I'm a bit confused and I wonder if you all could help me? How are you all feeling now?" (the affect focus). "What's it like to feel stuck like this? Some of these comments feel different from what I have heard from you all in previous sessions, especially when it comes to how much you do care at times for one another." Mom explains that the anxiety that comes with knowing Lydia is often alone with her pain and doesn't readily share with her is frightening. "Linda, I wonder if Lydia knows why you want to understand what she is going through so much. Can we ask Lydia?" Lydia indicates that she hasn't heard that from Mom and isn't sure Mom really cares, as when Mom does ask questions, it feels "fake." The therapist wonders with Mom if she has heard this before from Lydia and what it's like to hear this now. They are able to think more about how Mom comes across as "fake" by engaging in an activity where they learn more about how they each see one another from the outside (a feelings/doing game).

Disengaging from Non-mentalizing: Teleological Mode

Right now, Lydia is in what we call "prove-it" mode (also known as teleological mode) with most of her relationships. You have to prove you love her by talking, acting, listening, and being a certain way all the time (despite what she throws at you verbally or physically). She expects her friends to act a certain way in relationships. This ensures she knows they are trustworthy, and she checks regularly to make sure they are still her friends. We also see this mode at play in her parents' response to Lydia's distress. During a session, Lydia is discussing a distressing social situation from her day at school. She becomes tearful and becomes quiet when her father interrupts. Impatiently, he tells her to move forward, ignore the person, or just learn to get along with people. He indicates that it's the same with the family; if she would just get along and be a part of the family, everyone in the family would be happy.

Be quick to intervene here and be willing to call out the elephant in the room. Share your dilemma aloud…"Dad, can I stop you? I'm thinking I may have missed something and I really want to check with you. However, I feel I need to check in with Lydia. Can you help me? Do you know what may have happened with Lydia right then? She seems to have become quiet, and I think I see something coming out of her eyes [tears, obviously]. Can we check this out with her?" Dad is able to check this out, and Lydia indicates that her father doesn't really want to get to know her and blames her for everyone's problems. "Lydia, can we check that out with Dad? Dad, I wonder if you are interested in learning more about Lydia." Dad insists he is, but he "just doesn't know how to get to know her, especially when she stays in her room all the time." "Lydia, were you aware Dad felt this way? No? Well, what is it like to hear? I wonder if he might try again if we could rewind. What might you tell him to do if he were going to listen to you about this situation again?" Return later to Dad and wonder with Dad openly: "Dad, I'm sorry I had to interrupt you there. I think I missed how you were feeling when you heard Lydia struggling with this social situation" (the affect focus).

The Mentalizing Loop

The mentalizing loop is a "route map" for the therapist to identify non-mentalizing patterns, or loops, within the family, and a path forward for families to get themselves out of sometimes never-ending and often-hopeless loops [4]. When you feel you have enough data that point to a possible pattern of non-mentalizing, wonder aloud with the family if they might also NOTICE this pattern. In Lydia's family, the therapist asks for permission to interrupt: "Can we pause for a moment? I wonder if you all might see what I think I'm seeing here. Everyone talks at the same time, and the volume gets louder and louder. It makes me wonder if you feel understood or feel heard. How do you see it?" This CHECKING allows the family to wonder aloud if they see this happening in the "here and now." MENTALIZING THE MOMENT involves sitting with emotions and really understanding what it's like when everyone is talking at the same time. How do they imagine they get into this situation? What purpose does it serve? Do they each contribute something to the dynamic in a way? "What does it feel like when we are in this situation?" Make sure to spend time really appreciating what it's like for each person in the moment. Mark the mentalizing by contrasting what it feels like when they are in the loop and when they are not.

Throughout, think aloud with the family about whether they might see this pattern happen in other areas of family life (GENERALIZE). Lydia's family identify early-morning stress at times and at bedtime when everyone is talking and not listening. We help them generalize and be curious if they would like to CONSIDER CHANGING how things go in their family. The family therapist doesn't assume that the family even wants to change this pattern and even checks this out aloud. CHECKING happens throughout the entire process, as we want to reinforce/mark mentalizing as the family considers the loop. The family is invited to NAME this loop and to do so in a clever way so that when the family or any one member identifies that they are in the loop, the phrase can be said aloud, which helps everyone (hopefully) return to the "mentalized moment" and remember their plan to do something different. The family is challenged to think together about how to describe "everyone talking at the same time." They come up with clever ideas such as "system overload," "family feud," and "no ears in the room, just mouths." We support the family in MENTALIZING THE MOMENT when they reflect on what it feels like when everyone is talking at the same time. How did they get here, and what is behind this behavior for everyone? "Let's really think about what it feels like to be in this loop right now. This will help us better recognize these moments in the future." INVITE VISION within the system by asking them if they could imagine a world where they are able to have conversations in which they really hear one another and feel heard. What would they each be doing differently? This would be a way for the family to get their own mentalizing online and know what to do when they are not mentalizing. They then take what they have learned in the session about slowing down, being curious, rewinding, and implementing these skills, and plan in the moment at home together.

You will see that the loop flows in no particular order, and the therapist might wander off and explore various family dynamics and other interactions and then return to the loop. In addition, the therapist can reinforce areas of mentalizing that need to be strengthened (identified in formulation) as the loop is co-constructed with the family. The goal is for the dialogue to move from a specific interaction and work toward "widening the lens" and "capturing more general understandings" related to this observation [5]. We will now examine several examples of loops and how they help the family members make sense of themselves (Fig. 3.2).

Fig. 3.2 The mentalizing loop

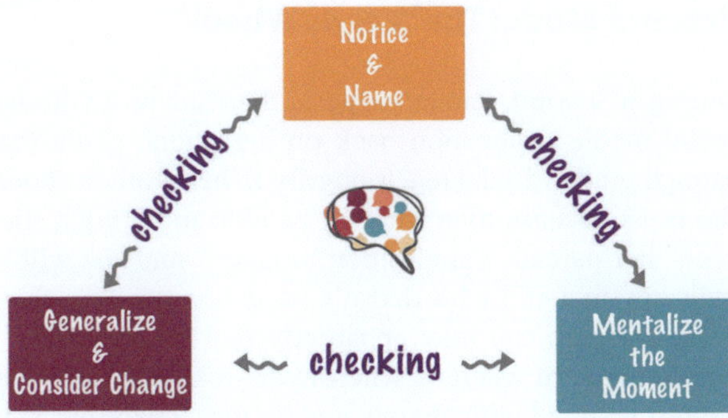

Psychic Equivalence: "Open Door?"

Lydia comes into a session tearful because her mother took away her phone last night. Mom indicates that Lydia came home "in a huff" from a school event and refused to talk. She took her phone because Lydia was "disrespectful" when Mom inquired about how she was doing. Because Lydia has refused to talk with her, she has become more certain that something bad happened and that Lydia had plans to hurt herself last night. Lydia indicates that the conversation lasted over an hour, with her Mom assuming all kinds of things, and they got nowhere because Mom wouldn't just give her space. As the therapist works to rewind what happened, he NOTICES a familiar pattern whereby Mom really wants to know what is in Lydia's mind, but does so quite intrusively and escalates to coercion. Thinking aloud, the therapist wonders if this feels familiar. The therapist supports them in MENTALZING THE MOMENT. Lydia indicates that her mother thinks the doors to both her room and her mind are open 24 hours. Slowing down (with much support!), Mom explains that the more she is learning about what is going on in her daughter's mind, the more she wants to know so she can be helpful. Tearfully, Mom shares that the idea of Lydia feeling so alone with her thoughts and maybe hurting herself to cope is scary and painful, and she really only wants to help her, not be hurtful. She can see that she asks a lot of questions, which is intrusive. Lydia is able to share that she wonders if her Mom really cares about her in these moments because she seems so focused on controlling Lydia's behavior. Mom indicates that when her daughter shuts her out, she feels helpless and alone. Lydia acknowledges these feelings as well, especially after blow-ups. They discuss other situations where Mom tends to feel like the door is always open. Lydia is able to discuss how actually Mom's anxiety only leads to more stress and isolation from the family. She can also appreciate how her silence may lead Mom to wonder about her. They become curious and are able to check out assumptions and misunderstandings. They are able to NAME this familiar pattern as "Open Door?" and are able to consider a world (INVITE VISION) in which Lydia and Mom are able to navigate the balance of privacy and open communication, especially in times of high emotionality. They are able to GENERALIZE other moments when this loop happens in their relationship (or even within the context of other relationships they each have), and they leave the session feeling prepared to identify and stop these patterns without the presence of the therapist.

Pretend Mode: The "Ferris Wheel"

During a session, Linda suggests that maybe Lydia isn't ready to have a certain social media application back on her phone given that she isn't achieving good enough grades. Lydia reacts angrily to her mother, shouting that she can't wait until she is 18 because then she will be able to do what she wants to do. She "doesn't need" her parents, "grades don't matter," and she will be "fine" on her own. Mom indicates that if Lydia doesn't need her parents, she will take away the phone because Lydia can now apparently pay for it herself. The therapist NOTICES a familiar pattern whereby when Lydia dismisses her need for parental support, her parents respond with anxiety and, in turn, coercion. The therapist wonders aloud if the family members recognize this pattern. It seems that when Lydia feels that someone is limiting her freedom, she makes comments about not needing others, which activates her mother's anxiety. Mom reacts quickly and joins Lydia in her pretend mode rather than responding in a more mentalizing fashion. The therapist shares the example of a "Ferris wheel" where they seem to go around and around and struggle to know how or when to get off. Through the process of MENTALIZING THE MOMENT, Lydia discusses how she is aware that she struggles to ask for help and accept help, but has a hard time conceding that she needs others. She becomes "stubborn" from her perspective and won't back down. Mom jokingly indicates that she might get this from her, as she also sees herself as "stubborn." Mom concedes that it's also hard to watch her only daughter get older, and she will try to give her more independence as they build trust with one another. They are able to consider other familiar situations in which they have been on this Ferris wheel (NAME) and neither of them could get off due to their stubbornness (GENERALIZE). Lydia reports that she does need help with some of her subjects but doesn't really know how to ask for it. She also wonders if it might make things worse if she asks for help. The family members are able to brainstorm ways of getting off the ride (CONSIDER CHANGE) and imagine what it would be like if they were quickly able to notice the Ferris wheel in the moment and do something different (INVITING VISION).

Teleological Mode: "Lecture Voice"

Lydia becomes deregulated in a session where she discusses a situation where a friend "broke her trust." Her parents quickly jump in, suggesting various things for her to do to manage the situation. Lydia becomes even more tearful and the therapist pauses, NOTICING the familiar pattern from the previous session where Dad jumped in and missed her and the opportunity to learn more about her. The therapist again does a rewind and comments on this possible pattern. The therapist wonders aloud if at times it's difficult for the parents to hear her distress with social situations and know how to help her. The parents acknowledge their anxiety and helplessness. Lydia is able to help her parents understand the importance of having space to just talk about her emotions when she is upset. She indicates that her parents tend to go into "Lecture Voice" rather than listen actively. The therapist wonders if they can sit in the moment with what it feels like to be in Lecture Voice. What do they each do, feel, and think? How do they look or come across to one another? By slowing down and MENTALIZING THE MOMENT, Lydia and parents are able to put into words their internal mental states and acknowledge they want to do something different (CONSIDER CHANGE). The parents want to be helpful and Lydia wants to open up about her feelings related to social issues with her parents. They are able to think about ways to pause when each of them is experiencing a moment of Lecture Voice and what they would do differently (NAMING). The therapist then encourages them to think about other times when Lecture Voice comes out (GENERALIZE) so they might be able to prepare for these as they leave the session. The therapist then will INVITE VISION by having the family explore what this might be like if they were able to unwind Lecture Voice situations before they become overwhelming.

Conclusion

As we have seen in Lydia's family, it's not just Lydia who struggles with mentalizing. Non-mentalizing is contagious and can spread like a wildfire, especially when it comes to the safety of our kids. Shame spirals can consume and dampen any sense of openness, curiosity, and willingness. Coerciveness in parenting styles can often be understood as desperate efforts to keep loved ones safe. This illusion of control comes at a cost, as it can breed mistrust and distance in relationships with children who are already struggling to feel connected. In session, the family learns from the mentalizing therapist the importance of slowing down, questioning oneself in the face of certainty, and being willing to go into conversations with an attitude that they may learn something new about one another. They learn to identify what others are feeling, learn to trust and share their own minds openly, and as a family learn to identify and address maladaptive patterns in the moment.

Lydia hasn't been sure that others in her family really care about her or even know her. Self-injury has been her way to really show, signal, and prove to her parents that she is in pain. With support and over time, Lydia learns more about what she does that gets in the way of her feeling heard and having her needs met, while her parents learn more about how their efforts to keep Lydia safe may result in Lydia feeling even more alone, isolated, and desperate. I have learned to recognize (and still work to trust this idea) that one of the most powerful tools I have as a therapist is my relationship with my clients. Mentalizing theory and techniques can allow a therapist to build trust with each family member in order to slow down and utilize active explicit mentalizing to promote agency and change within the family system.

Lydia and her family have struggled to comprehend one another, especially in times of intense emotionality and increased risks of suicidality and self-injury. This family—like many that are struggling with suicidal thoughts and actions, and self-injurious, dysregulated behavior—has been in these cycles for years. Using the mentalizing toolbox allows all family members to own their 2%, more clearly see themselves from the outside and others from the inside, name non-mentalizing moments, and together build new processes for change in the face of intense emotional storms. Indeed, as they use these tools outside their sessions, the emotional storms and self-injury/non-suicidal self-injury (SI/NSSI) gradually improve. What we are shooting for is more than a happy ending. It's a curious series of endings, over and over again, with each understood misunderstanding making the next more likely! We considered naming the mentalization-based treatment for families (MBT-F) loop the "virtuous cycle," but evidently that name was already taken.

Supporting the family in re-establishing a sense of security within the context of the family system, when nothing feels safe for them, requires much work from those in the family system. For the therapist, it's important to keep the mentalizing raft available at all times. For me, I stay afloat because of my consult groups, supervision, personal therapy, self-care, mentors, family, and willingness to talk openly about my own fears and struggles as a therapist. It is when I feel mentalized in these ways by these supports that I do my best mentalizing as a therapist.

References

1. Fonagy P, Gergely G, Jurist EL, Target M. Affect regulation, mentalization, and the development of the self. 1st ed. New York: Other Press; 2002.
2. Yalom ID. The theory and practice of group psychotherapy. 4th ed. New York: Basic Books; 1995.
3. Bateman A, Fonagy P. Handbook of mentalizing in mental health practice. 1st ed. Arlington: American Psychiatric Publishing; 2012.
4. Asen E, Fonagy P. Mentalization-based therapeutic interventions for families. J Fam Ther. 2012;34:347–70.
5. Bateman A, Fonagy P. Handbook of mentalizing in mental health practice. 2nd ed. Washington, DC: American Psychiatric Publishing; 2019.

4 Mentalization-Based Treatment Activities, Games, and Intersession Activities

Chris W. Grimes and Laurel L. Williams

Introduction

The focus of this chapter is to provide some specific activities that might help promote mentalizing. Mentalizing is fundamentally an ACTIVE activity. Understandably, for a book about suicidal and self-harming youth, we have not yet emphasized how much fun can be had with mentalization-based treatment for adolescents (MBT-A). We will now rectify that deficit! We often explicitly discuss *mentalizing* (the verb) versus *mentalization* (the noun) in order to focus the minds of the therapist and the person on action. As we noted in Chap. 2, a mentalizing therapist is on the edge of their seat, engaged in the active back and forth necessary to maintain the mentalizing balance. For a mentalizing therapist who is monitoring the mentalizing temperature of the session, activities can assist in moving from a too-cold session (pretend mode) or a too-hot session (teleological mode or psychic equivalence) back into balance. Additionally, activities can also assist a therapist in better understanding the mentalizing abilities of the patient and family members [1]. Since we know it is normal for all people to turn mentalizing off and on both globally and with specific subject matter, an activity can assist you and the participants to procedurally notice, mark, and name a non-mentalizing hotspot. Importantly, for families and therapists, the kinds of activities that promote mentalizing share a quality with humor: imagining and misunderstanding minds, and then working out what we got wrong, can be fun. This is why jokes are funny—"Oh, I thought there was going to be another answer to why the chicken crossed the road! But the answer is simpler than I could have imagined!" Similarly, getting curious and active is significantly more fun than therapy that feels like a refereed boxing match. So prepare to be a big hit with families when you utilize the following activities!

C. W. Grimes · L. L. Williams (✉)
Menninger Department of Psychiatry and Behavioral Sciences, Baylor College of Medicine, Houston, TX, USA
e-mail: laurelw@bcm.edu

L. L. Williams, O. Muir (eds.), *Adolescent Suicide and Self-Injury*,
https://doi.org/10.1007/978-3-030-42875-4_4

Mentalizing therapists are mindful of words and their meaning, relentlessly seeking to engage in improved understanding. To that end, we are sensitive to the idea that a word activity or game may appear to be too "lighthearted" when suicide or self-injurious thoughts or behaviors are being discussed and worked through. However, it is this exact dilemma that we ask you the therapist to ponder. Recall that in Chap. 1 we discussed how infants learn about their minds. Is it through the parent screaming at them or when they scream at their parent? No, dear reader: it is when the parent brings forth the *marked mirroring behavior* repertoire. When do humans learn? They learn when their secure base is activated and generally when an environment is conducive to feeling safe. So we encourage you, a mentalizing therapist, to assist in modeling why an activity or game becomes essential in the quest for improved mentalizing skills.

Such activities promote structure, safety, and playfulness around exploring mental states [2]. Their very playfulness and inherent humor is part of the built-in challenge that makes such activities work so well in restoring mentalizing. Activities provide emotional distance, safety, and predictability, which is more likely to bring mentalizing online and restores epistemic trust within the context of the attachment relationship. Once epistemic trust is restored, families are able to think about one another, to learn new aspects of themselves and their family members, to discuss unspoken concerns or feelings, and hence to understand misunderstandings. These types of interactions become important opportunities for all members of the family to practice skills such as distress tolerance, emotion regulation, interpersonal effectiveness, and mindfulness. In general, activities allow members to see themselves from the outside and others from the inside, and hopefully find the process meaningful and enjoyable.

We will provide the reader with six specific mentalizing activities that a therapist might consider employing to restore the balance such that oneself and others can be better understood and misunderstandings can be replaced with improved awareness. As we discuss each of these activities, we will review with the reader what elements make an activity mentalizing. It is our contention that you will discover or invent many additional activities that will assist a young person, a family, or a group once you have in mind the action of mentalizing. We also wish to clarify that many of these maneuvers may feel familiar to more seasoned therapists. This, too, is by design, as when an activity enhances understanding of oneself and others, it bolsters mentalizing. As you read this chapter, consider what activities you may already be successfully engaged in. Do they promote mentalizing? If yes, that's wonderful. If not, consider whether these activities would become even more successful if they were changed to more directly emphasize mentalizing. There is one simple maxim to bear in mind: keep things surprising!

This chapter will discuss the following

1. Introducing the other
2. The pause button
3. Inverted roles
4. Feeling and doing
5. Family modeling
6. The mind [or brain] scan
7. Indications for and timing of activities

Introducing the Other (Introduction, a Challenge for Pretend Mode)

"Introducing the other" is a mentalizing icebreaker for getting to know the family while also introducing the family to the mentalizing stance. This type of activity can be your first foray into mentalizing with the patient and their family as you do an initial assessment. This activity is also useful if/when a new person comes to a session or group for the first time. As you will learn in Chap. 6 of this book, you can even use this type of activity to encourage participants to consider someone who is not presently in the room in order to better define the social connections your patient or family may have within a mentalizing context.

Family members are encouraged to spend time introducing one another to the therapist; that is, the youngest person introduces the next youngest, and so forth. The question "Can you tell me about _____?" is fairly wide open initially to allow the person to say what comes to their mind. Encourage them to take time as they consider their introduction. Prompting is fine if the person is feeling anxious, overwhelmed, or shy, or feels "stuck." Recognize that you might be putting them on the spot, and be curious about what they are thinking. If a prompt is needed, approach the person by suggesting "I'm wondering if you are feeling stuck, and I wonder if other members might know what might be getting in the way. Can I ask a few more questions to help out, if you like?" You can prompt them by having them think about who the person is, what kind of Dad/Mom/sister/brother they are, and how they feel when they are around the person.

If the process feels safe for the family (and we might wonder this out loud), you might expand on the questions by having each family member reflect on the introduction—for instance, "What was it like to hear her describe you in this way to me? How did it feel? Did she leave something out? Are you surprised by something that was said?" At the end of the activity, the family members reflect on how they were introduced by each other, and each introduced family member members reflect on introduction and whether it "fits" what they know about themselves, what was it like to be introduced, and so forth. The "circular" nature of this process (perspective, checking, revision of perspective, checking, repeat) is of course part of the model called the *mentalizing loop*, which was discussed in Chap. 2.

In this activity the therapist begins to assess the individual and family capacity to mentalize, noting specific mentalizing strengths and non-mentalizing modes. Family members can also learn quickly that what they think or could have imagined was in another family member's mind, or what they "know" about one another, is not always the case, challenging certainty. Often we may hear members describe family members in very concrete terms or really struggle with finding words to describe the other person. They may focus on roles or, behaviors, or make assumptions. They may leave out the "negative" qualities of the other or, alternatively, focus very much on what is wrong.

This activity provides a sense of scaffolding and safety for the young person as they realize that the intervention is aimed at supporting the family, not particularly focused on intruding into "just" the young person's mind. The family is introduced immediately to new ways of being and interacting with one another. The family learns how the mind of the therapist works and begins to trust the space provided. This lays the groundwork for the family to have future conversations including the specific topic of suicide and self-injury.

The Pause Button (a Challenge for Psychic Equivalence or Teleological Mode)

This is a maneuver that requires some preparation before utilization. Indeed, you might want to consider bringing this forward as an essential ingredient in mentalizing therapy when you introduce the shared "rules" for creating a safe place. As always, your modeling of using a "pause button" will further reinforce the concept as a key component of improved mentalization.

Using clay, a patient or their family will create a pause button of their own. The therapist supports the building and personalization of the pause button. The therapist explains that the pause button is a physical representation (not all teleological things are bad) that provides a reminder that each of them has the power to slow down and do something different. I often use the example of a "time-out" in basketball. When things are not going as anticipated, the coach may call a time-out. This provides a breather, time to regroup, and an opportunity to do something different when the time-out is over. I reinforce the fact that the game continues after the time-out and the importance of coming back to the non-mentalizing moment to repair. When mentalizing in this way, the family members each become willing to step back, pause, mentalize, and come back in a more curious and intentional way the next time around. Just being able to slow down provides opportunities for mentalizing to come back online, supporting mentalizing moments, emotion regulation, and agency [2]. Those of you who are familiar with improvisational comedy will recognize this pretty quickly; it's almost identical to the game "freeze," with the pauses being used for therapeutic instead of comedic effect.

The pause button gives everyone the opportunity to slow down rather than react. For instance, it could be really important for everyone to slow down when the young person might be struggling and signaling the need for support. Recognize that this is not the easiest thing to do for anyone in these moments. A simple (or not so simple) push of the pause button provides an opportunity to slow down. Pausing ensures for the adolescent that parents might slow down and provide him/her with the right amount of space and consider new, ideally more helpful ways of responding. Discuss moments when the family successfully paused during the week when a familiar loop or emotional state arose. It can also be powerful to reflect on moments in which the pause button could have been pushed. Recall how often this device has been used by playwrights—the pause and "aside" as the character breaks the fourth wall to explain their mental state to the audience before returning to the interactions with the other characters! This is exactly what we want the family to be able to do: stop the "non-mentalizing" train of the current heated exchange and reveal their thoughts and feelings in a momentary aside in which the pressure to keep fighting is put on pause!

The therapist can also push their pause button during sessions, having the family freeze in moments when the therapist identifies moments of non-mentalizing or good mentalizing [1]. Typically, I find that most adolescents/parents utilize the pause button when they feel misunderstood or are finding others incomprehensible. This activity provides the family with the opportunity to imagine what each individual is feeling and thinking, and to get clarity in playful ways: "I'd like to check that out with you."

Variations of this activity might include brainstorming other "button" ideas. For instance, the family might develop a "volume control button" that anyone can turn up or down, depending on the temperature of the conversation. The family may develop a "curiosity button," allowing any member to push it when there is a lack of curiosity in the room. Explain that there are also times when you might turn that button off and turn a "listen button" on. These buttons allow the family to focus on the areas of mentalizing that can be strengthened and give everyone a sense that they can have an impact on the interaction. These buttons are ways for the family to practice mentalizing in the moment and consider new ways of doing things.

Inverted Roles Activity (All Three Mentalizing Failures)

As described by Asen and Fonagy, inverted roles activity is designed to engage the family in "seeing that other people have difficulties, too, and that they might be able to help with finding a solution" [2]. The therapist has the family members switch roles and guide one another/navigate a specific situation or interaction. As in psychodrama, the role-reversal technique provides a way for the individual to really put themselves in the shoes of another person. To start, the young person identifies a situation for the parents to be in. Through this activity, the young person becomes privy to what the parents would be thinking, feeling, and doing if they were in the situation. At some point, the therapist encourages the parents and young person to reflect on the activity and how they think and feel in both similar and different ways [2]. The parents can also come up with situations for the young person, who will take on the role of the parents, while the parents play the young person.

For example, a young person struggling with medication compliance might take on the role of the parent charged with ensuring that the young person is taking the medication, while the parent takes on the role of the young person not taking their medication. In another example related to self-injury, a young person might take on the role of his father, who comes in and finds his son cutting himself. He must respond to this situation and in doing so has to put himself in the shoes of his father. The father, playing the son, will imagine what it's like to be the young person being confronted. For the son to put himself in the shoes of his father can be a powerful discussion as well.

Asen and Fonagy observe that "the therapist's main role is to facilitate the role-play and subsequently encourage family members to reflect on their own and others' experiences, with the aim of appreciating both the similarities and the differences of one another's minds" [2]. To make things more playful, the therapist can take on the role of the "director" of the activity, who can slow them down or cut to another moment, while supporting the mentalizing process. This activity provides the family members with practice in perspective-taking and curiosity, and challenges certainty. What they think they would do if they were the person isn't always what comes out as they role-play. They may also be jolted out of pretend mode by really working through what they would do in the situation. When in teleological mode, or "prove-it" mode, the families learn there are likely multiple ways of addressing a problem rather than anyone having to "prove" themselves. Rather, we support discussions around what it might be like to trust and be trustworthy, especially when things are not going well or feeling safe.

The "Feeling and Doing" Activity (Pretend Mode)

As described by Asen and Fonagy, the "feeling and doing" activity provides an opportunity for the family to explore "how different people respond to their inner feelings" [1]. The therapist has each family member discuss various emotions they have experienced in the context of the family over the past week. These emotions may include protective, confused, concerned, happy, angry, etc. The therapist encourages the family members to think about hot/cold emotions. After six to eight emotions are identified, the therapist, who participates actively in the game, asks everyone to imitate (without mocking) one particular emotion displayed by a family member (e.g., rolling eyes when irritated) and also to state what other family members do when they feel irritated. The family then engages in the game "hot potato" [2]. One person throws the potato (or ball) and names one of the emotions mentioned above. The catcher then acts out how the thrower acts when experiencing the emotion. The catcher becomes the thrower and the game continues. The therapist encourages the family to go faster and faster until the therapist pushes the pause button.

As Asen and Fonagy explain, "The therapist asks what this was like for each person during the activity, and the family then discusses how different and similar they are in how they express emotions" [2]. This activity allows the family members to reflect on emotional responses in themselves and each other. Ideally, the family members learn more clearly how to support and respond to one another based on more accurate readings of the other person. The therapist takes the opportunity to explore the feeling states more, continuing to model the mentalizing stance.

Other variations may include the thrower stating an emotion and the catcher responding with a moment in the past week when they felt the emotion in the context of their relationship. The thrower may mention an experience or situation and the catcher will state what he or she felt in that situation. The thrower may call out an emotion and the catcher will display what they look like when they feel that way [2].

Family Modeling (Pretend Mode, General Lack of Knowledge)

Family modeling activity allows all members to practice representing family dynamics and individual feeling states in a visual representation. This allows the family members to explore how they experience one another, and to have a way of looking at themselves from the perspectives of another. Have the family consider, either together as a group or individually, how they might represent themselves and family members if they were the artist. This could be anything from a depiction of what the family might look like in the middle of one of their loops or a representation of a recent moment of non-mentalizing. You might have the family create a model using one another and items/space in the room (similar to family sculpting in psychodrama), and support one member in explaining his "artwork" to the rest of the family.

The therapist prompts the family with questions focusing on affect, perspective-taking, and impact awareness. The family members explore what they each look like from the outside and what others might imagine the other person is feeling and thinking on the inside. For instance, what's it like for Mom to have to hold everyone together? What's it like being the lost child, so far away from the rest of the family? I wonder why all the negative energy is going towards Dad. *You can also have them recreate the family model, but in ways they want the family to look like*—for instance, in a circle with more togetherness rather than distance.

For Lydia's family, whom we discussed in Chap. 3, Lydia models her family with Dad going in and out of the door, with her and her mother pulling each other's hair, and with her brother with a laptop in the corner by himself. This image allows the family to really imagine what the world looks like from Lydia's perspective. Dad is able to sit with Lydia's view that he is in and out, and becomes curious about what this is like for her and the rest of the family. Mom is tearful and discusses with Lydia's brother whether he feels this way. Lydia uses her magic wand to show the family how she wants it to be. They all sit in a circle and play a family game of cards together.

The Mind [or Brain] Scan (Pretend Mode; General Lack of Mentalizing)

The *mind scan* (or *brain scan*) [1] is an activity that allows members to really think about what is in the mind of another (Fig. 4.1). The therapist gives a diagram of a brain (Fig. 4.1) to each family member. Each family member wonders what might be in the mind of the other person and fills in the circles with thoughts/feelings the other person might be having around a specific topic or situation, and preferably in the moment. The other person fills out what is actually in their mind, and this is followed by a discussion. This activity illuminates for the family the limits of mind reading and how often we do not really know what is in another's mind [2].

Lydia and her Mom spend time completing the brain scan activity after a blow-up in a session about Mom going through Lydia's room and finding razor blades. They each fill out a brain scan of the other brain. Each is asked to think about what the other is feeling and thinking after the blow-up. Mom imagines that her daughter hates her and will never talk to her again. Lydia indicates that she imagines that Mom will never trust her again and never give her space. They are both able to talk about what they are feeling and check out what really might be going on for each of them.

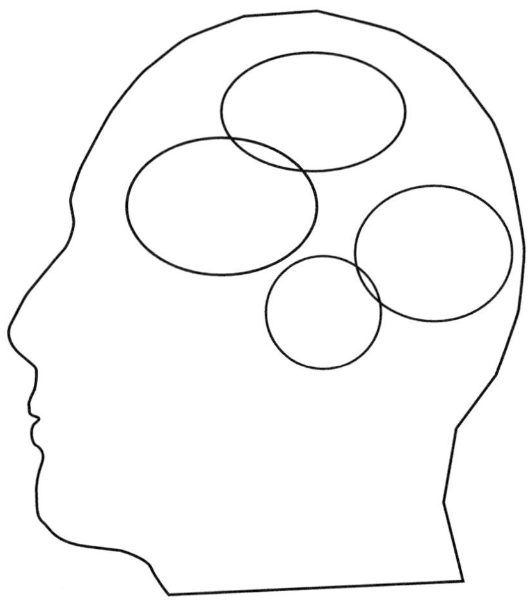

Fig. 4.1 The mind scan [or brain scan]. (Reproduced with permission from the Anna Freud Centre for Children and Families)

There are many variations of this activity with the goal of exploring the thoughts/feelings of oneself and others, challenging possibly strongly held beliefs about one another. Asen and Fonagy note that "The therapist can support the family in speculating about how the brain might have looked before a specific event or how it might or should look in 6 months' time" [2].

Safety, Timing, and Communicating About Games/Activities

The mentalizing therapist strives to keep in mind what it's like for each member of the family to engage in playful ways in the midst of serious issues. Assume and be explicit that it's not always easy to be vulnerable, especially in the context of family, and check out what it might be like for the family to be playful. The mentalizing therapist will appreciate what it might be like for each member and ask for permission, while providing a clear explanation of the game/activity and the intent behind the intervention. How will this be helpful to the family, and why am I deciding to implement this tool right now? Monitoring arousal of emotional states during these activities is important in order to not overwhelm the family system. Encourage members to speak up if they are feeling uncomfortable and share this aloud. In addition, activities can bring about a lot of emotions for everyone, and you want to check in and support the family members as they transition to the end of the session. Also, at times, families need games to actually warm things up if the therapist has a concern about overall inhibition of emotional expression.

Mentalizing activities can be a nice start to subsequent sessions. More structured activities might be planned ahead, and maybe you can even have the family consider thinking about how they might implement the family sculpting activity for the following week. The willingness of each family member is crucial for activities to be an effective mentalizing tool. Much of knowing what will work and if it's safe is your connection with and active mentalizing of the family. As you develop a mentalizing formulation, dear reader, you can start to envision which activities may help address specific mentalizing difficulties you consider are present.

Modeling the Mentalizing Stance, Playfulness, Humility, and Use of Humor

The mentalizing stance remains the therapist's "compass" [3] throughout sessions. Holding the balance, terminating non-mentalizing interactions, marking good mentalizing, and remaining curious/not knowing are imperative. There are multiple members to hold in mind during sessions, and you must acknowledge that you will likely miss something. Encourage the family to let you know if they are feeling on the spot or left out, for instance. Monitor for non-mentalizing and mark mentalizing as you engage in activities. You might use the pause button at times to "pause" the family and have them consider what it's like for each family member in the moment. As mentalizing clinicians, we naturally strive to understand what it's like to really do this work from the other side of the couch. We can only know by mentalizing clients and working hard to create an environment where families feel safe and understood.

As you try out any of the activities discussed here, or develop your own (as we strongly encourage you to do), do so in a mentalizing manner. What would be most helpful to this family right now? Can they tolerate the emotions this activity might evoke? Can they really be playful about this subject right now? Will the game help them actually talk about things, in a playful way, that might otherwise feel overwhelming? Might it be more of a distraction rather than helpful? Why am I employing this activity? If an activity really seems to not be working out (as has happened many times for me), this may be an opportunity for a mentalizing moment. Own for yourself the fact that the game didn't turn out as planned. This provides more security in the sessions for others to make mistakes and feel free to "bumble around" [4]. The idea that there might be "do-overs" when mistakes are made can be reinforced in these mentalizing moments.

Family members have told me that some of the more powerful mentalizing moments have come during moments of humility, playfulness, and humor shared as a family. Monitor how families and therapists use humor to avoid falling into non-mentalizing family interactions. Some clients are the ones everyone enjoys poking fun at, and we might even imagine that this person enjoys it, depending on their reaction. Take these moments to check in and consider feeling states, and be willing to use these as ways to model mentalizing moments.

Troubleshooting Avoidance of Games

At times, games/activities may feel clinically appropriate but the family is quite reluctant and really struggles with being playful. Acknowledge that this might be difficult, and wonder with the family if another style could be appropriate for them. What did they imagine could be helpful? This provides an opportunity to understand what it's like for you to have an idea but for it not to fit with how they would like to do things. I would reinforce that I think these games might be helpful but understand their perspective. You can always return to the games/activities in the future. If they are willing to give it a chance, you can always come back to it.

Conclusion

Mentalizing activities allow for families to talk and think about difficult, anxiety-provoking, and scary topics while approaching one another in not-so-serious, playful ways. Games provide a relaxed atmosphere and one that takes families out of their usual ways of interacting. Mentalizing activities support the therapy process and support openness, problem-solving, flexibility, and willingness to learn from one another. We encourage creativity in the process of creating games as well as using those described here. You can find more games in the *Handbook of Mentalizing in Mental Health Practice* [2].

References

1. Asen E, Fonagy P. Mentalization-based therapeutic interventions for families. J Fam Ther. 2012;34:347–70.
2. Asen E, Fonagy P. Mentalization-based family therapy. In: Bateman A, Fonagy P, editors. Handbook of mentalizing in mental health practice. 1st ed. Arlington: American Psychiatric Publishing; 2012. p. 107–28.
3. Allen JG, Bleiberg E, Haslam-Hopwood T. Mentalizing as a compass for treatment (white paper). Houston: The Menninger Clinic; 2003. http://citeseerx.ist.psu.edu/viewdoc/download?doi=10.1.1.461.7525&rep=rep1&type=pdf.
4. Epictetus. The art of living: the classical manual on virtue, happiness, and effectiveness (trans: Lebell S). New York: Harper Collins; 1995. In: Allen JG, Fonagy P, Bateman AW, editors. Mentalizing in clinical practice. 1st ed. Arlington: American Psychiatric Publishing; 2008. p. 182.

Suicidality in Context

5

Carl Fleisher

Introduction

An array of mental illnesses are linked to suicide, suicide attempts, and non-suicidal self-injury (NSSI). For brevity we will use *suicidality* as an umbrella concept for these three behaviors, unless there is a specific distinction to highlight for the reader. Why are so many diagnoses linked to suicidality? Some risk arises directly from the diagnosis, as in depression. Some risk of suicidality is common across diagnoses or, in other words, transdiagnostic. This chapter discusses both illness-specific and transdiagnostic contributions to the risk of suicidality, divided into five areas: trauma, personality pathology, internalizing symptoms, externalizing symptoms, and general health.

At the end of this chapter, you, dear reader, will:

1. Understand how trauma and specific mental illnesses impair mentalizing, thereby increasing the risk of suicidality
2. Understand how failures of mentalizing may, in turn, impact specific mental illnesses
3. Consider how skills learned in this chapter may help address mentalizing failures and therefore suicidality in youth

Childhood Trauma

We address childhood trauma first because it is the predominant transdiagnostic risk factor for suicidality. Trauma is transdiagnostic because it confers later vulnerability to a wide array of psychopathology, including all of the problems discussed later in this chapter. Trauma is also transdiagnostic in its effects on attachment and on

C. Fleisher (✉)
Psychiatry and Biobehavioral Sciences, University of California, Los Angeles, Los Angeles, CA, USA
e-mail: drcarl@drcarlfleisher.com

L. L. Williams, O. Muir (eds.), *Adolescent Suicide and Self-Injury*,
https://doi.org/10.1007/978-3-030-42875-4_5

mentalizing—effects that can occur even in the absence of formal psychopathology. In this chapter, we narrow our consideration of trauma down to abuse and neglect—here referred to collectively as *maltreatment*—though we also discuss bullying as a trauma of particular importance in adolescence [1].

Maltreatment Disrupts Mentalizing, Attachment, and Trust

Maltreatment impairs mentalizing: no one in the midst of being maltreated is able to contemplate why perpetrators do what they do—nor should they. Moreover, maltreatment is especially harmful to mentalizing when perpetrated by a family member, in comparison with maltreatment by someone outside the family [2]. Intrafamilial maltreatment is probably worse because it sends the message that someone I inherently should be able to trust considers me to be "worthless" or needing punishment. And, since that person is trusted, the worthlessness will seem true. At the same time, it is impossible to imagine how a trusted person could see a child in that way. As a result, mentalizing becomes disrupted, certainly for that relationship and potentially in other attachment relationships as well. In this way, the concept of the *alien self* discussed in Chap. 1 perhaps becomes more alive: maltreatment, such as telling a child they are "worthless," becomes internalized even though it is not an authentic part of the self. For some, this inauthentic part becomes the driver first of self-hatred and then, in extremes, of suicidal actions. The reader will recall from earlier chapters in this book that mentalizing fosters children's self-esteem and agency. When maltreatment inhibits mentalizing, it reduces self-esteem and agency broadly. If the damage is sufficient, children may sink to feeling self-loathing and helplessness. Vulnerability to such feelings may result in suicidality, regardless of the diagnosis; this is what makes maltreatment a transdiagnostic risk factor.

Maltreatment disrupts attachment, which may also result in suicidality. Attachment is fundamentally a mechanism for security, so maltreatment damages children's sense that someone will keep them safe. When children are highly distressed, they have a natural, hardwired urge to seek out an attachment figure. If an attachment figure has also perpetrated maltreatment, that distress leaves children seeking comfort from the very person who has hurt them. While the attachment figure may indeed provide comfort at times, at other times the child's need may overwhelm or aggravate the attachment figure, potentially provoking further maltreatment. As Jon Allen [3] and others have eloquently noted, the essence of trauma is feeling not merely afraid but both *afraid and alone* (p. 163). This aloneness explains the finding that the risk of developing posttraumatic stress disorder (PTSD) after trauma is greatest not with a particular type of trauma but when a person who was traumatized gets no reaction, or gets a critical one, from the people to whom they are most attached. There is no aloneness more profound or more pernicious than when a child suffers maltreatment at the hands of an attachment figure. A child, maltreated and alone, might understandably deteriorate to despair and suicidality.

Importantly, impaired mentalizing has itself been shown to be a transdiagnostic risk factor for suicidality [4]. Maltreatment leads to emotion dysregulation [5, 6]. When mentalizing—the means of self-understanding—is limited by maltreatment, children will have difficulty labeling, and communicating, their emotions. Thus, they are likely to be, and feel, misunderstood more easily. When misunderstood, children's distress can spiral and become overwhelming. Overwhelmed youth can act out, engaging in risky behavior or suicidality. Hence, just as maltreatment can increase the risk of suicidality directly by disrupting self-esteem and agency, it also raises the risk indirectly via impaired mentalizing, insecure attachment, and emotion dysregulation.

The effect of maltreatment on insecure attachment, can carry forward into adult relationships and parenting, leading to intergenerational effects. Berthelot and colleagues [7] found that when mothers had a history of childhood maltreatment, their ability to mentalize had a measurable impact on their children's attachment style. For mothers who were never maltreated, mentalizing did not affect attachment. Mothers who have been maltreated also have high rates of disorganized attachment, which is a risk factor for PTSD among children later exposed to trauma [8]. Maltreatment, then, by increasing the risk of unhealthy attachment, and also by increasing the risk of PTSD, can increase young people's risk of suicidality.

How Can Therapists Work Productively with Youth Who Have Suffered Maltreatment?

Fortunately, just as mentalizing can be impaired by maltreatment, the experience of being mentalized by a therapist can repair some of the damage caused by such trauma. Since maltreatment has varied effects, as noted above, several types of opportunities may arise in therapy.

Recall that mentalizing allows for the epistemic trust superhighway to form. In later chapters in this book, you will hear more about the highway either being completely closed off, in a hypervigilant style, or too porous, both of which create problems for whether youth will accept input from you as a helping professional. If a young person's epistemic trust system is malfunctioning ("their guard is up," as it were), then new information and new attachments will struggle to take hold. Therapists can begin by naming this difficulty with trust, making it something that is at least acknowledged, as well as shared, and making distrustful youth feel seen and less alone. Once difficulty with trust is recognized, the work is to develop a greater understanding of its components. What makes someone trustworthy, or not? How is that gleaned from interaction, from conversation? How does one decide how much of oneself to share? What tells a youth how their sharing is being perceived? Does sharing engage the other person, or turn them off, or outright scare them? Conversely, how does a lack of sharing come across? Is it appropriate to that type and stage of relationship? Does it leave behind an opportunity to connect with someone? And if disconnection is preferred despite the cost (loneliness), what makes that worthwhile?

These questions are numerous, yet vital. Youth who have never been maltreated may comfortably navigate between implicit and explicit management of these questions; a typical example would be talking with a romantic partner about whether to see each other exclusively. Those with a history of maltreatment, on the other hand, may be unable to bring these questions to explicit attention without guidance and support. Instead, they might at times act in relationships entirely unaware of this level of relating to others, controlled by their reflexive (mis)trust and attachment reactions.

One common example of the effects of trauma is seen in youth who haven't learned to understand their own and others' emotions. They will concretely struggle to put their experiences into words, especially when it comes to an attachment figure. This is recognizable when a young person, asked (for example) for her or his reaction to a difficult family situation, says, "I don't know." Hearing that, therapists who know their clients well may be tempted to supply the answer, to substitute their understanding for that of the client: "Oh, you *must* have felt …" jumps too easily off the tongue. A mentalizing intervention, however, would be first to consider what "I don't know" means. Does it signal genuine confusion, or reluctance to be honest, or pretend mode, or something else? With this healthy uncertainty in mind, therapists can then assist youth in finding their own words to describe their reactions, their needs, or their goals. "How was that for you?" one might say, or "What were your needs at that time?" or "What went into feeling overwhelmed?" or, most simply, "I am not sure I know what you mean. It seems really important that I understand you—can you say more?"

A second common situation is when youth claim to understand themselves, or others, yet do not. These pseudo explanations are identifiable as "too [something]": too black-and-white ("She hates me"), too paranoid ("He doesn't really like me; he's just using me"), too simple ("I'm just sad"; people typically have many reasons for any given reaction or decision), too vague ("My parents won't let me go because they're too busy worrying about my sister"), or too external ("Those are just the rules"). Such statements may fall under psychic equivalence, if discussed with high emotional temperature, or under pretend mode, if discussed with little to no emotional temperature. Here, therapists should not take initial explanations, however plausible, at face value. Instead, it is more fruitful to probe what lies beneath (a strategy outlined in Chap. 2 for pretend mode), making sure to empathize with whatever emotions are encountered. This approach, when genuinely curious, will stimulate mentalizing and foster trust, in place of (inappropriate) certainty and misunderstanding.

Bullying

Bullying can be traumatic and drive youth to suicidality [9]. Bullying has such an impact because, as youth pass through their school-age years, their self-esteem depends increasingly on the opinions of their peers—a process that peaks in adolescence. Though victims of bullying are certainly at risk of suicidality and psychopathology, research shows that the youth at greatest risk are those who are both victims and also perpetrators of bullying [10]. Such youth are termed bully–victims. Bully–victims are often viewed by peers and adults solely as bullies, as people who need punishment rather than assistance. This is a failure to mentalize bully–victims that may reduce their sense of belonging to a peer group, adding further risk of suicidality.

Bullying and victimhood are each indicative of impaired mentalizing [11]. Bully youth resort to acting out (i.e., teleological mode) when they cannot describe, or when they get overwhelmed by, their needs or feelings. In younger children, disagreement about who gets to play first with a toy may provoke aggression; in older children, unmentalized internal needs (e.g., for attention or importance) may cause anger or shame that lead to bullying. Victimized youth may have other mentalizing deficits—for example, making socially awkward comments or crying instead of being able to problem solve. Being in a social minority (arbitrarily or otherwise [12]), or being socially marginalized (e.g., lesbian/gay/bisexual/transgender/queer (LGBTQ) youth), further increases one's chance of victimhood. Though bullying may be verbal or physical at early ages, for adolescents it is largely verbal. All bullying carries a subtext of exclusion, of course. Exclusion is painful and is a direct risk factor for suicidality [13]. Some bullies may even explicitly tell victims to kill themselves.

To repair poor self-esteem caused by bullying, we can address peer interactions. Self-esteem and agency reinforce one another, so therapeutic interventions that bolster agency directly, that help youth state what they need with words rather than attacking or retreating, are ideal. Victimized youth who successfully challenge bullies, who act in ways that lead bullies to back down, will enjoy greater self-esteem. Self-esteem will improve in part because youth can then see themselves as more agentive, as capable of changing how others treat them. Bullies equally will need help expressing their needs with polite words rather than vicious ones. They may even need help knowing what they need (i.e., mentalizing themselves).

What does this work look like? The starting point would be seeking an understanding of the situation(s) that trigger bullying, whether for a victim or for a perpetrator. Therapists may work with victimized youth to help them decide on confident or even friendly[1] things to say to bullies. These might include direct responses like "I'm sorry you feel that way," deflecting responses such as "Hmmm, OK," or non-sequiturs like "That's a cool shirt you're wearing; where'd you get it?" Therapists working with bullies and bully–victims may help youth sort out how to go to a counselor to say, "I argued with my parents this morning" instead of lashing out at peers.

Bullies' ability to harm others requires a deactivation of empathy and, more fundamentally, of mentalizing. Thus, any of the mentalizing techniques described in this book are potentially useful to help victims fend off bullies. Interventions like the non-sequitur example above would be akin to a challenge in mentalization-based treatment. Saying "I'm sorry you feel that way" is an example of affect focus. Statements that make the relationship between bully and victim explicit may reactivate mentalizing, and empathy, in the bully. When mentalizing is active, violence or verbal abuse becomes more difficult to carry out.

Mentalizing interventions targeting teachers and schools are also effective responses to bullying. A large study by Fonagy, Twemlow, and colleagues [11] evaluated an intervention across an entire school district. The researchers educated teachers and staff about mentalizing, emotion regulation, and power dynamics. They found reduced aggression and improved classroom behavior. This effect was significant, over and above an active comparison intervention, suggesting that a focus on mentalizing adds something that may be lacking in standard bullying

[1] see https://www.brooksgibbs.com/320396. Accessed 6 May 2019.

interventions. Children in schools that received this mentalizing intervention for two or more years even showed improved academic performance ([13, 14], personal communication, October 2018).

While maltreatment and other forms of trauma such as bullying are pervasive, a host of other insults, external and internal, heighten the risk of suicidality in youth. A full consideration of those is beyond the scope of this chapter, but issues of particular relevance are detailed below.

Personality Factors

Borderline Personality Disorder

Borderline personality disorder (BPD) in adolescents is clearly associated with increased risk of suicide attempts and NSSI [15]. In some studies, the percentages of youth with BPD who have been found to engage in such behavior have been 75% or greater [16]. NSSI is, of course, included in the very definition of the disorder, underscoring the close relation between the two [17]. Youth with BPD frequently also have a history of trauma, further heightening the risk of suicidality [18]. As the reader can, hopefully, see, BPD is the disorder at the intersection of major predisposing factors for suicidality (maltreatment and impaired mentalizing).

In a mentalizing framework, the suicidality seen among youth with BPD is understood as arising out of impaired mentalizing. The first step in this process is that threats to attachment relationships (real or perceived) cause intense emotional arousal. Arousal of that intensity inherently disrupts mentalizing, giving way to non-mentalizing—be it psychic equivalence, teleological mode, or pretend mode. If the former two are present (as they often are together), youth may be convinced that suicidal behavior of one kind or another is the only viable method of either managing or communicating the seriousness of their feelings. Pretend mode—which can happen as a result of, or sometimes before, NSSI—may be even more dangerous. In pretend mode, youth who normally would not attempt suicide (because of how their family would feel, for example) may be so emotionally disconnected that this barrier vanishes. They may carry out more serious self-harm than they otherwise would.

Mentalizing therapy for BPD is always aimed at helping the client feel seen and understood; no progress can be made without that. For youth with BPD, distress seems as if it comes "out of nowhere," yet inevitably, it can be linked to something. That something is usually an interpersonal interaction, typically one involving some sort of attachment (i.e., romantic or care giving) relationship. Clear empathy is the crucial first step. Therapists should be prepared to take youths' distress at face value, no matter how outlandish a client's perception of events may seem. The stance here is as if one were sitting down for coffee with a friend, delivering empathy unquestioningly. ("Oh, how terrible!" is adequate, for example, as long as it is genuine.) Once an empathic statement is made, the therapist can begin to clarify the client's experience. Use brief, probing questions such as "How was that for you?" or "What was your reaction?" or "What did you make of that?" This type of exploration provides both a deeper sense of empathy (therapists who ask may want to understand) and helps youth recover mentalizing, at least as it pertains to themselves. Once the therapist sees glimpses of mentalizing, she or he can encourage youth to generate alternative perspectives on the situation—reverting to empathy if those attempts evoke non-mentalized responses.

Narcissism

Narcissism and narcissistic personality disorder (NPD) have also been associated with either a higher likelihood of suicide attempts or greater lethality of attempts [19–23]. People with pathological narcissistic traits tend to be prone to attempt suicide following occupational failures, rather than interpersonal ones as would be typical in BPD. Ansell and colleagues [23] found that people who met the criteria for NPD had the greatest likelihood of making more than one suicide attempt, even accounting for the presence of BPD. An inability to regulate shame may drive this vulnerability [24]. At the same time, other studies have shown no increase in suicidality among people with narcissistic traits or have even found a protective effect of those traits [25, 26]. These seemingly opposing findings may be explained by the fact that people with NPD usually avoid suicidality because of grandiosity and their characteristic low impulsivity. On the other hand, during acute distress, people with narcissistic pathology may experience so much shame that they reach the point of suicidality. They may make more numerous and more lethal attempts because of their greater ability to plan and carry out actions, relative to people with BPD.

When treating youth with pathological narcissism, resist any temptations either to be critical of their need for admiration or to be secretive, as if clients were too fragile to hear their insecurities spoken aloud. Rather, we encourage the reader to put the pathology "on the table" as a focus of treatment. People rarely have trouble acknowledging their desire for attention and admiration, which at that age is normal to a certain extent (and something all of us wish for in some quantity). Thus, therapists can raise the topic without hesitation. For example, "It seems like it really bugs you when you don't have everyone's attention" would be one mild approach.

Ensure the client is aware of the link between this desire for admiration and their behaviors when that is lacking. "How do you react when others are perceived as [better in any way]?" we can ask. Youth with adaptive narcissism may respond by working harder, achieving more, or creating new and useful things. When narcissism is excessive, however, the lack of admiration can lead youth to substance use, suicidality, or risky behavior (especially when they are intoxicated). These behaviors may be reinforced sometimes by the attention they garner, though at other times they may be off-putting to peers, unfortunately exacerbating the lack of attention or admiration.

Another approach to narcissism is to mentalize—that is, to discuss explictly—what feelings are generated by a lack of attention, which then drive unhealthy behaviors. Here, again, the point is to assist youth in mentalizing their own mental states, rather than mentalize for them. Hence, asking "How is it for you when you feel you don't have enough attention?" is preferable to a seemingly innocent yet leading question like "Does not being noticed enough make you feel like you don't exist?" Though youths' feelings are often some predictable version of shame or nothingness, it is premature to assume so, or to assume that we know how feeling shame (or any other feeling) will affect someone. As clients practice awareness of those feelings, we anticipate the feelings will become easier to tolerate.

Antisocial Personality Disorder

Suicidality has been associated with psychopathy [27]. Since most research in this area involves adults with antisocial personality disorder (ASPD) or with antisocial traits, here we will extrapolate from that population to youth with conduct disorder. People with ASPD organize their lives around dominance and hierarchical relationships—highly teleological arrangements. When dominance is threatened, feeling "weak" or "lesser" is intolerable and typically drives aggression, but it may drive suicidality. There are other facets of ASPD that compound this risk: impulsivity, a vulnerability to negative emotional responses, and a low fear response. Although some authors have suggested that the increased risk of suicidality among people with ASPD is wholly accounted for by co-morbid BPD [28], others have found links between suicidality, ASPD, and co-morbid NPD, independent of BPD [22, 29]. Interestingly, one study of military personnel found that people who scored highly for antisocial traits were likely to express low desire for suicide yet had strong plans to carry it out [13]. The authors of that study concluded that people with antisocial traits also may be more likely to use talk of suicide for secondary gain.

Therapists who work in juvenile justice, or more generally with boys who are aggressive, are likely to encounter youth with this type of pathology. (Of course, girls and women can be antisocial and aggressive, but they are in the minority and attract much less clinical attention.) How can therapists address the risk of suicidality, or the threat thereof, among such clients? People with antisocial traits have difficulty mentalizing emotions in themselves. With that in mind, any treatment intended to reduce the risk of suicidality should be aimed at improving mentalizing of self.

A prime target for a mentalizing intervention is the vulnerability to negative emotional responses seen in ASPD. Improving youths' mentalizing of their self-states may allow them to feel understood, soothing those negative emotions. Linking situations to reactions may help with this goal. Helpful questions could include "What made you feel that way?" or "What happened that made you feel that way?" Often it can clarify things to ask, "What about [the situation] caused that sort of feeling?" When clients feel understood, it generally lessens the chance they will act on negative emotions.

A second target might be improving youths' awareness of their sensitivity to hierarchies—that is, of how upsetting it is not to be dominant or in charge. Feeling understood in this way might also lessen their reactions. One way to do this, since anger will frequently be expressed, is to help youth look "behind the curtain" at what is driving their anger. Are they feeling humiliated, ashamed, powerless, unimportant, afraid, or something else? How can they describe it? Many youth will not want to admit such feelings, but they may tolerate hearing the therapist talk about them: "Gosh, if I felt it was so important to be [in charge, the strongest] and someone did that to me, I might feel almost humiliated!" In building awareness of these emotions, youth begin to tolerate them; the more emotions are felt and tolerated, the less they need to be acted on.

Internalizing Disorders

Mood and Anxiety

Mood disorders—bipolar or unipolar depression—and anxiety obviously confer a risk of suicidality [30]. Suicidality may arise directly, as in the throes of depression, or indirectly, as when a manic state is ending. Youth with anxiety may become suicidal if they anticipate or experience great embarrassment, if they feel judged and alone, or if they become too narrowly pessimistic about the future. In addition, trauma and personality pathology make coping with mood and anxiety episodes more difficult [31]. People with co-morbid mood and personality disorders show more mood lability, making it harder to define the onset and offset of mood episodes [32]. When depression seems to have no beginning nor end, youth may more readily become hopeless, then suicidal. Mood lability may also be off-putting to friends or others who form a client's support network; less support also increases one's risk of suicide.

Psychic equivalence, in depression, takes the form of hopelessness, guilt, and suicidality. The mentalizing therapist who targets these has several opportunities. The first will be empathizing with the depth of emotion—for example, "It's just awful to be [betrayed by your friends]!" Note that the validation used here is absolute: it *is* awful that the youth *has been* betrayed. Empathizing with someone's view as a fact rather than a perception helps it come across effectively, but empathy should still be marked, to convey that the therapist is not overwhelmed. A second opportunity is to clarify that a range of feelings is present, then link feelings to events. For example, one might ask, "Is it just *sad* that you feel, or other emotions, too? What brought up those emotions?" After clarification reboots mentalizing, and not before, the therapist can try to help the client build an alternative perspective. Perspectives need not be hopeful, but simply different. They may be gathered from other people or from other times in the client's own life. Thus, a therapist might say, "Were you feeling suicidal like this yesterday? How come?" A non-mentalizing response to a question that offers perspective means that the client is not ready to see the situation a different way. Likely more empathy is needed, or a new topic, or possibly a challenge, before returning to entertaining other points of view.

Anxiety attacks (which youth may mislabel as "panic" attacks) are typically the height of non-mentalizing in anxiety disorders. They indicate psychic equivalence—that a threat is real, not perceived, and is serious. Therapists can generally use the approach described above with youth in this state. One important adaptation for anxiety, however, relates to when youth ask for reassurance. Although it is detrimental in the long term, giving reassurance may be appropriate in the service of restoring mentalizing. Another adaptation is that during anxiety attacks, non-mentalizing can be even more difficult to disrupt than it is in depression. Thus, it is helpful for therapists to have a strong (yet compassionate) challenge at the ready.

Pretend mode can be seen in youth caught up in depressive (or anxious) rumination. In this state, they are "overthinking"—that is, thinking without a genuine connection to their emotions or their present experience. The lack of a connection to real experience found in pretend mode means that anything, bad or good, is possible. This can be paralyzing because when the worst is possible, failure becomes inescapable and all solutions are discounted. Mentalizing therapists can guide youth who are ruminating toward their current, embodied experience. For example, one could pair an observation with a question: "I notice you seem to be going over and over the same thing in your mind right now. Can you tell me how you are feeling?" or "Instead of spinning our wheels [a subtle, compassionate challenge by using first-person *plural*], can we rewind to what we were talking about a few minutes ago?" Yet another alternative is to rewind to a time before pretend mode launched. "How did you get started on this?" one could ask.

Hopelessness can be the most difficult non-mentalizing state to disrupt. Youth who are hopeless often tempt the therapist into a self-reinforcing existential discussion—for example, by stating, "There is no point to living; we are all going to die eventually." This argument feels so weighty and morbid, it can evoke hopelessness in the therapist. But it is pretend—mere words. Proof of this comes in remembering that the argument could easily be flipped on its head; inevitable death could justify a hedonistic (prioritizing pleasure above all) approach, rather than a fatalistic one. To escape a pretend discussion, therapists must disengage from the content. Logical arguments will not convince clients. Instead, therapists will more probably have success using the mentalizing polarities: ask about affect and then link it to the "here and now" or rewind to a time when the client did not see life so darkly.

Disordered Eating

Suicidality is common among people with eating disorders (ED). The rate of suicide attempts among people with ED ranges from 20% to 33% [33]. NSSI is seen in up to 40% of youth with ED [33–35]. Among people with bulimia nervosa, NSSI has been associated with transient difficulties with emotion regulation [36]. Moreover, people with ED or a personality disorder sometimes engage in disordered eating as a method of NSSI. Suicidality and NSSI are important to address in their own right among youth with ED; when present, they also limit the success of family-based treatments [37]. This may arise in part because suicidality and NSSI negatively impact parents' caregiving experience [38].

Disordered eating may impact mentalizing in various ways. In general, as Pisetsky and colleagues [39] explain, "difficulties with identifying and understanding emotional states, as well as problems selecting adaptive over maladaptive emotion regulation strategies, are associated with cognitively-oriented global ED symptoms." Another effect is that disordered eating behavior itself arouses intense shame, making it even harder for youth to accurately imagine others' minds. Moreover, youth with severe anorexia nervosa may be so underweight that malnutrition limits their brain function, including mentalizing. Finally, if bingeing disrupts electrolyte balances, that too can impair mentalizing. When non-mentalizing takes hold, we view restricting, bingeing, purging, etc., as teleological efforts to escape feeling out of control or overwhelmed. Some research shows that mentalizing is impaired more among people with ED and NSSI than among people with ED alone [40]. Disordered eating and impaired mentalizing, then, may drive each other in a vicious cycle.

Studies investigating the risks of suicidality and NSSI among people with ED have also identified transdiagnostic factors linked to impaired mentalizing: childhood trauma/abuse, insecure attachment style, emotion dysregulation [41, 42], and co-morbid personality disorder [34]. In families of people with ED, for example, mothers' self-reported enmeshment—a characteristic of insecure attachment—accounted for nearly 40% of the variance in ED symptoms [43]. In addition, youth with co-morbid ED and BPD may engage in disordered eating to manage intense emotions.

Mentalizing interventions can help youth with ED. To address disordered eating, like other psychopathology, begin by slowing down and "rewinding." The aim is to identify a moment before a particular instance of disordered eating began, back when mentalizing was starting to deteriorate. Then, be curious—not about the disordered eating itself but, rather, about the events and emotions that led to thinking about food or body image in the first place. If youth are unsure, therapists may suggest themes common to ED—control, shame, and family—to see if those spur youth to notice and name their trail of emotions.

Therapists can also use mentalizing to help youth with body image; that is, therapists can encourage youth to connect what they see on their "outside" (in the mirror) to what they are like as a person on the inside. For example, restricting helps youth achieve a sense of control, which they struggle to find elsewhere in their turbulent lives. This reliance on action (don't eat) to change a mental state (out of control) indicates teleological mode. In these youth, teleological mode may actually short-circuit intense emotions rather than fuel high emotional arousal as one would see in BPD. Therapists' mentalizing interventions, then, will aim to upregulate emotional arousal. Therapists can ask youth what situation or feelings led to the urge to restrict at a particular moment. Youth may give concrete, external answers ("I looked fat") to these sorts of inquiries, so the therapist's challenge will be to push for internal experiences ("What was this like for you on the inside?"), taking care not to push too far and flood clients with emotions they can't manage. This can generate discussion that identifies interpersonal triggers, leading to more relational methods of coping.

Pretend mode is also found in ED. For example, a youth in pretend mode might acknowledge that disordered eating is present, yet maintain that everything she or he is doing is "fine" or "under control," with no acknowledgment of the risks involved. Any attempt to argue with, convince, or otherwise rationally approach youth about this is very likely to be ineffective. Instead, facing pretend mode, therapists are encouraged, as always, to probe for emotions, both "here and now" and when maladaptive behavior occurs. Therapists must be wary of allowing intellectualization or provocative statements by youth to distract therapists from discovering how they feel.

Externalizing Disorders

Substance Use Disorders

Substance use increases the risk of suicidality in youth [44, 45]. Recent cannabis use doubles the risk of a suicide attempt [46]. After using cannabis, men in one study had a greatly increased risk of self-injury [47]. In other studies, chronic cannabis use has been associated with an increase in the risk of suicide attempts [48]. The risk from other substances (e.g., benzodiazepines, cocaine, tobacco, alcohol) appears to be even greater than that conferred by the use of cannabis [49, 50]. Early initiation of substance use confers a greater risk of suicidality than later initiation [51]. Intoxication during a suicide attempt, as one might expect, is associated with a greater risk of completing suicide [52, 53].

Suicidality, in turn, predicts greater use of substances [54]. In one major population health study, for example, women with suicidal ideation were more likely to initiate cannabis use later on [47]. With youth, this author's experience shows that when low self-esteem leads to recurrent suicidality, they are more open to using any psychoactive substance that will mask their unhappiness for a time. Treatment of substance use disorders (e.g., methadone treatment for opiate use disorder) lowers people's risk of suicidality [55].

Substance use impairs mentalizing in multiple ways. Not only does intoxication directly impact self-awareness, other-awareness, and judgment, but also the overall process of addiction hijacks the brain's attachment network, which, as noted earlier, is a hardwired link to mentalizing [56, 57]. New mothers with substance use disorders, for instance, show impaired mentalizing of their infants [58, 59]. The overlap between addiction and attachment suggests that people with substance use disorders may have difficulty mentalizing when in the throes of cravings or withdrawal, or while going through a relationship problem, wholly apart from the effects of intoxication.

How could mentalizing therapy lower the risk of suicidality among youth struggling with substance use? Use and relapse are related to interpersonal triggers at times and also to automatic, overlearned processes like cravings. Increasing mentalizing of self could give youth a healthier approach to interpersonal relationships, certainly, or more control over their reactions to cravings. Other opportunities arise in the light of the significant co-morbidity between personality disorders and substance use disorders. Some research has shown that negative emotionality is more important than impulsivity in understanding substance use, when a personality disorder is co-morbid [60]. This finding suggests that strengthening mentalizing, as a buffer against negative emotionality, may lower the risk of suicidality even when impulsivity persists. In a longitudinal study, personality pathology was shown to precede substance use disorder [61]. Hence, addressing mentalizing deficits associated with personality disorders may help prevent deterioration of substance use, and its associated risk of suicidality, into a full-blown disorder.

Substance misuse itself can be viewed as a manifestation of non-mentalizing, of teleological mode. When youth are overwhelmed, they may believe that the only way to survive that experience is to *do* something to the mind, to manipulate it chemically. Psychic equivalence typically drives that teleological response, as when feelings (shame, anger, or any others) become so strong that they are experienced as facts. Feelings that strong cannot be held at a distance for consideration and cannot be balanced or juxtaposed against other perspectives; instead, they must be extinguished, as with drugs or alcohol, lest they grow too painful.

When substance misuse is seen in the light of non-mentalizing, the reader may see how coping skills, or even acknowledging a higher power, can fall short. A mentalizing intervention, in this case, would start with empathy. To then reassert mentalizing, the therapist can ask the youth to travel back in their memory to before the episode of substance use, to a situation where mentalizing was near baseline—was only beginning to fade from view. This might be on the same day, or in the same hour, as the substance use, or it might be on the day before. "When did you *start* to think about getting high?" one would ask. Or, more directly, "What shifted your thinking from making social plans to getting hammered?" The purpose of such questions is to maintain mentalizing in session, by jointly focusing on a past time when the youth was mentalizing, even if transitioning out of it. *In contrast, asking youth to analyze a situation where mentalizing was already lost will generally just foster more non-mentalizing.*

Non-mentalizing can also be present when discussing sobriety. Whether youth say they plan to quit using substances, or that there is nothing wrong with their use, both can reflect pretend mode. Telltale signs would be if therapists feel that youth are "just saying what adults want to hear" or, in contrast, that youth are "living in their own world." In these instances, a mentalizing intervention will look a lot like motivational interviewing (MI). In MI, therapists first focus on understanding clients' reality (i.e., using the mentalizing skills of empathy and clarification). They build trust and reduce defensiveness by asking in detail about substance use, acknowledging the benefits that clients get from it. After some trust is established, but not before, youth may be encouraged to consider alternative perspectives, such as a therapist nudging them to also describe the downsides of substance use. That description must also be from the client's point of view in order to sustain empathy.

General Health and Social Factors

Insomnia

Persistent insomnia is frequent in youth and increases the risk of suicide, independent of co-morbid psychiatric illness ([62, 63]; see McCall and Black [64] for a review). Not surprisingly, people whose insomnia is co-morbid with BPD or chronic pain are at particularly high risk [65]. Investigations of suicidality in insomnia have been framed using the interpersonal theory of suicide [13]. This theory posits that suicide results from a combination of three factors: thwarted belongingness, perceived burdensomeness, and capability. In this model, insomnia may indirectly lead to thwarted belongingness via its impact on daytime function [66].

Insomnia's many detrimental effects—impaired judgment, irritability, and hopelessness—may cause and result in mentalizing failures that underlie poor daytime function. Youth with insomnia and hopelessness may be less motivated to socialize; those with irritability may socialize less effectively. Notably, insomnia in youth is often caused by anxiety, compounded by dysfunctional (e.g., pessimistic or passive) beliefs about sleep [65]. This combination of factors suggests a role for mentalizing interventions in treating insomnia to reduce suicide risk.

Youth may talk about insomnia in pretend mode, making comments such as "I know this is a problem, I can fix it if I just…." (As noted in earlier chapters, the phrases "I know…" and "just" indicate pretend mode.) When encountering pretend mode, focus on emotion: "Does the insomnia bother you? How?" is a simple inquiry. Alternatively, one can ask, "When bedtime comes, what keeps you from doing [simple solution] or [adaptive behavior]?" and "How does it feel to do [sleep-interfering behavior]?" Questions about emotion tend to highlight competing or inconsistent priorities, since youth may acknowledge strong emotions related to insomnia, yet avoid confronting them, and describe insomnia as a low priority.

Psychic equivalence and teleological mode can perpetuate insomnia in the moment, even if they are absent in a therapy session. Youth will say they "need to" do whatever bedtime-interfering behavior they do (e.g., browsing social media or using cannabidiol). Here, as usual, therapists will want to elicit and empathize with whatever feeling(s) drive non-mentalizing. If that fails, asking youth to keep a journal or to try a mindfulness exercise at bedtime may create an opportunity for them to notice their emotions clearly enough to then describe them. When empathy does land effectively, therapists may be able to explore and clarify which daytime stressors (short- or long-term) lead to the feelings at bedtime. This process of linking emotions to events eventually helps youth tolerate emotions. With time, they can choose healthier coping behaviors or even regulate their bedtime emotions on their own.

Chronic Medical Illness and Somatic Symptom and Related Disorders

Chronic medical illness is associated with a higher risk of suicidality. Singhal and colleagues [67] found elevated rates of NSSI among adults with seven illnesses: asthma, epilepsy, migraine, psoriasis, diabetes mellitus, eczema, and inflammatory joint disease (see also Tietjen and colleagues regarding migraine [68] and Singh and colleagues regarding psoriasis [69]). Three of these—asthma, eczema, and migraine—are relatively common in youth. Similar findings have been reported regarding chronic fatigue syndrome [70, 71], chronic pain [72–74], gastric cancer [75], and cancer in general [76]. Remarkably, in a study seeking to distinguish suicide completers from attempters, Giner and colleagues [19] found that health problems were second only to the presence of NPD as a predictor of completion.

Given the impact of physical illness on suicidality, one might wonder whether perceived illness—i.e., somatic symptom disorders—would have a similar effect. Riem and colleagues [77] studied adults with a variety of "medically unexplained somatic symptoms." They found correlations between somatic symptoms, anxious attachment, and low levels of mentalizing (i.e., emotion awareness). Bizzi and colleagues [78] studied youth with similar pathology. They found high rates of disorganized attachment (~50%), which was associated with poor mentalizing in a clinical group compared with healthy controls. One study even suggested a connection to BPD: they found that people with BPD described higher levels of fatigue and pain than those with other forms of psychopathology [79]. As we have seen in earlier sections of this chapter, impaired mentalizing, disrupted attachment, and BPD are indeed strong risk factors for suicidality. What might explain why impaired mentalizing is associated with both physical and psychosomatic illnesses? The reader will recall that mentalizing oneself is a physical, embodied process of reading internal signals—analogous to reading body language in other people. For youth who misread their internal signals, then, it will come as no surprise that a risk of suicide co-exists with medical or psychosomatic illness.

This difficulty may be heightened among survivors of maltreatment. Maltreatment could interfere with psychological development to the extent that some children would mainly be aware of distress in its physical form. Alternatively, maltreatment might interfere with physical development to make children misinterpret, or be hypersensitive to, their internal states. Further, there are biological pathways by which trauma can increase vulnerability to medical illness (collectively termed *toxic stress* [80]). Changes in inflammation, stress hormones, and gene expression may all play a role. Consistent with a toxic stress model, Post, Altshuler, and colleagues [81] found that adults with bipolar disorder who reported a greater number of adverse childhood experiences had an increased risk of eleven different medical conditions, including allergies, menstrual/uterine irregularities, fibromyalgia, and irritable bowel syndrome.

How can mentalizing therapists work with this population of youth? Medical and psychosomatic symptoms seem closely associated with non-mentalizing in the form of pretend mode. Therapists likely need to help youth develop greater emotional awareness, by asking detailed questions about their reactions to events. Therapists can also encourage clients to pay close attention to the situation(s) *leading up to* the physical symptoms. This might allow clients to notice previously missed emotional reactions that come before, or at the same time as, physical reactions. As clients develop greater real-time awareness of their internal world, we expect the intensity and frequency of their physical symptoms to diminish. Of note, therapists should avoid the temptation to suggest that clients' physical symptoms are merely a bodily manifestation of emotion (i.e., "It's all in your head"). First, that is inaccurate, and second, it runs the risk of further exacerbating clients' pretend mode. Indeed, when the *Diagnostic and Statistical Manual of Mental Disorders, Fifth Edition* (DSM-5) was published in 2013 [17], it shifted the emphasis in somatic symptom disorders away from a concept of feigned or imagined symptoms to a concept of excessive and undue distress about physical symptoms—regardless of what causes them.

Conclusion

This chapter has reviewed how trauma, mental illness, and physical illness can impact youths' suicidality, both directly and indirectly. All of these conditions disrupt mentalizing, putting youth in a state of mind where hopelessness reigns unchallenged (pretend mode), where social exclusion is absolute (psychic equivalence), or where suicide or non-suicidal self-injury seems the only way to communicate one's pain to others (teleological mode). This makes mentalizing a shared (i.e., transdiagnostic) link from symptoms to suicidality. The other primary transdiagnostic risk factor for suicidality is maltreatment. Maltreatment derails the developmental process whereby being mentalized by an attachment figure builds self-esteem and agency. Absent those capacities, people find it difficult to trust others and to build relationships. Diminished trust thus leaves people alone, psychologically or literally, and hence at greater risk of suicide and non-suicidal self-injury. The mentalizing techniques suggested herein aim to reduce suicide risk directly, by addressing non-mentalizing, as well as indirectly, by enhancing the effectiveness of treatments across a wide range of psychopathology.

References

1. Koyanagi A, Oh H, Carvalho AF, Smith L, Haro JM, Vancampfort D, et al. Bullying victimization and suicide attempt among adolescents aged 12–15 years from 48 countries. J Am Acad Child Adolesc Psychiatry. 2019;58(9):907–18.e4.
2. Ensink K, Normandin L, Target M, Fonagy P, Sabourin S, Berthelot N. Mentalization in children and mothers in the context of trauma: an initial study of the validity of the Child Reflective Functioning Scale. Br J Dev Psychol. 2015;33(2):203–17.
3. Allen JG. Mentalizing in the development and treatment of attachment trauma. New York: Routledge; 2013.
4. Navarro-Haro MV, Wessman I, Botella C, García-Palacios A. The role of emotion regulation strategies and dissociation in non-suicidal self-injury for women with borderline personality disorder and comorbid eating disorder. Compr Psychiatry. 2015;63:123–30.
5. Serafini G, Canepa G, Adavastro G, Nebbia J, Belvederi Murri M, Erbuto D, et al. The relationship between childhood maltreatment and non-suicidal self-injury: a systematic review. Front Psych. 2017;8:149.
6. Titelius EN, Cook E, Spas J, Orchowski L, Kivisto K, O'Brien KHM, et al. Emotion dysregulation mediates the relationship between child maltreatment and non-suicidal self-injury. J Aggress Maltreat Trauma. 2018;27(3):323–31.
7. Berthelot N, Paccalet T, Gilbert E, Moreau I, Merette C, Gingras N, et al. Childhood abuse and neglect may induce deficits in cognitive precursors of psychosis in high-risk children. J Psychiatry Neurosci. 2015;40(5):336–43.
8. MacDonald HZ, Beeghly M, Grant-Knight W, Augustyn M, Woods RW, Cabral H, et al. Longitudinal association between infant disorganized attachment and childhood posttraumatic stress symptoms [Erratum in Dev Psychopathol. 2008;20(4):1351]. Dev Psychopathol. 2008;20(2):493–508.
9. Barzilay S, Brunstein Klomek A, Apter A, Carli V, Wasserman C, Hadlaczky G, et al. Bullying victimization and suicide ideation and behavior among adolescents in Europe: a 10-country study. J Adolesc Health. 2017;61(2):179–86.
10. Winsper C, Hall J, Strauss VY, Wolke D. Aetiological pathways to borderline personality disorder symptoms in early adolescence: childhood dysregulated behaviour, maladaptive parenting and bully victimisation. Borderline Personal Disord Emot Dysregul. 2017;4:10.

11. Fonagy P, Twemlow SW, Vernberg EM, Nelson JM, Dill EJ, Little TD, et al. A cluster randomized controlled trial of child-focused psychiatric consultation and a school systems–focused intervention to reduce aggression. J Child Psychol Psychiatry. 2009;50(5):607–16.
12. Bloom S. Lesson of a lifetime. Smithsonian Magazine. https://www.smithsonianmag.com/science-nature/lesson-of-a-lifetime-72754306/. Accessed 6 May 2019.
13. Chu C, Buchman-Schmitt JM, Stanley IH, Hom MA, Tucker RP, Hagan CR, et al. The interpersonal theory of suicide: a systematic review and meta-analysis of a decade of cross-national research. Psychol Bull. 2017;143(12):1313–45.
14. Fonagy P, Twemlow SW, Vernberg E, Sacco FC, Little TD. Creating a peaceful school learning environment: the impact of an antibullying program on educational attainment in elementary schools. Med Sci Monit. 2005;11(7):CR317–25.
15. Reas DL, Pedersen G, Karterud S, Rø Ø. Self-harm and suicidal behavior in borderline personality disorder with and without bulimia nervosa. J Consult Clin Psychol. 2015;83(3):643–8.
16. Goodman M, Tomas IA, Temes CM, Fitzmaurice GM, Aguirre BA, Zanarini MC. Suicide attempts and self-injurious behaviours in adolescent and adult patients with borderline personality disorder. Personal Ment Health. 2017;11(3):157–63.
17. American Psychiatric Association. Diagnostic and statistical manual of mental disorders, fifth edition: American Psychiatric Association; 2013.
18. Kaplan C, Tarlow N, Stewart JG, Aguirre B, Galen G, Auerbach RP. Borderline personality disorder in youth: the prospective impact of child abuse on non-suicidal self-injury and suicidality. Compr Psychiatry. 2016;71:86–94.
19. Giner L, Blasco-Fontecilla H, Mercedes Perez-Rodriguez M, Garcia-Nieto R, Giner J, Guija JA, et al. Personality disorders and health problems distinguish suicide attempters from completers in a direct comparison. J Affect Disord. 2013;151(2):474–83.
20. Pincus AL, Ansell EB, Pimentel CA, Cain NM, Wright AGC, Levy KN. Initial construction and validation of the Pathological Narcissism Inventory. Psychol Assess. 2009;21(3):365–79.
21. Heisel MJ, Links PS, Conn D, van Reekum R, Flett GL. Narcissistic personality and vulnerability to late-life suicidality. Am J Geriatr Psychiatry. 2007;15(9):734–41.
22. Blasco-Fontecilla H, Baca-Garcia E, Dervic K, Perez-Rodriguez MM, Lopez-Castroman J, Saiz-Ruiz J, et al. Specific features of suicidal behavior in patients with narcissistic personality disorder. J Clin Psychiatry. 2009;70:1583–7.
23. Ansell EB, Wright AGC, Markowitz JC, Sanislow CA, Hopwood CJ, Zanarini MC, et al. Personality disorder risk factors for suicide attempts over 10 years of follow-up. Personal Disord. 2015;6(2):161–7.
24. Jaksic N, Marcinko D, Skocic Hanzek M, Rebernjak B, Ogrodniczuk JS. Experience of shame mediates the relationship between pathological narcissism and suicidal ideation in psychiatric outpatients. J Clin Psychol. 2017;73(12):1670–81.
25. Coleman D, Lawrence R, Parekh A, Galfalvy H, Blasco-Fontecilla H, Brent DA, et al. Narcissistic personality disorder and suicidal behavior in mood disorders. J Psychiatr Res. 2017;85:24–8.
26. Cross D, Westen D, Bradley B. Personality subtypes of adolescents who attempt suicide. J Nerv Ment Dis. 2011;199(10):750–6.
27. Harrop TM, Preston OC, Khazem LR, Anestis MD, Junearick R, Green BA, et al. Dark traits and suicide: associations between psychopathy, narcissism, and components of the interpersonal–psychological theory of suicide. J Abnorm Psychol. 2017;126(7):928–38.
28. McGonigal P, Harris L, Guzman-Holst C, Martin J, Clark H, Morgan T, et al. Is suicidal behavior in antisocial personality disorder better accounted for by comorbid borderline personality disorder? Poster presented at the Annual Meeting of the Association for Behavioral and Cognitive Therapies; San Diego; 16–19 Nov 2017.
29. Douglas KS, Lilienfeld SO, Skeem JL, Poythress NG, Edens JF, Patrick CJ. Relation of antisocial and psychopathic traits to suicide-related behavior among offenders. Law Hum Behav. 2008;32(6):511–25.
30. De Crescenzo F, Serra G, Maisto F, Uchida M, Woodworth H, Casini MP, et al. Suicide attempts in juvenile bipolar versus major depressive disorders: systematic review and meta-analysis. J Am Acad Child Adolesc Psychiatry. 2017;56(10):825–831.e3.

31. Post RM, Altshuler LL, Kupka R, McElroy SL, Frye MA, Rowe M, et al. Verbal abuse, like physical and sexual abuse, in childhood is associated with an earlier onset and more difficult course of bipolar disorder. Bipolar Disord. 2015;17(3):323–30.
32. Kopala-Sibley DC, Zuroff DC, Russell JJ, Moskowitz DS, Paris J. Understanding heterogeneity in borderline personality disorder: differences in affective reactivity explained by the traits of dependency and self-criticism. J Abnorm Psychol. 2012;121(3):680–91.
33. Kostro K, Lerman JB, Attia E. The current status of suicide and self-injury in eating disorders: a narrative review. J Eat Disord. 2014;2:19.
34. Islam MA, Steiger H, Jimenez-Murcia S, Israel M, Granero R, Agüera Z, et al. Non-suicidal self-injury in different eating disorder types: relevance of personality traits and gender. Eur Eat Disord Rev. 2015;23(6):553–60.
35. Peebles R, Wilson JL, Lock JD. Self-injury in adolescents with eating disorders: correlates and provider bias. J Adolesc Health. 2011;48(3):310–3.
36. Muehlenkamp JJ, Engel SG, Wadeson A, Crosby RD, Wonderlich SA, Simonich H, et al. Emotional states preceding and following acts of non-suicidal self-injury in bulimia nervosa patients. Behav Res Ther. 2009;47(1):83–7.
37. Downs KJ, Blow A. A substantive and methodological review of family-based treatment for eating disorders: the last 25 years of research. J Fam Therapy. 2013;35(Suppl 1):3–28.
38. Depestele L, Lemmens GM, Dierckx E, Baetens I, Schoevaerts K, Claes L. The role of non-suicidal self-injury and binge-eating/purging behaviours in the caregiving experience among mothers and fathers of adolescents with eating disorders. Eur Eat Disord Rev. 2016;24(3):257–60.
39. Pisetsky EM, Haynos AF, Lavender JM, Crow SJ, Peterson CB. Associations between emotion regulation difficulties, eating disorder symptoms, non-suicidal self-injury, and suicide attempts in a heterogeneous eating disorder sample. Compr Psychiatry. 2017;73:143–50.
40. Cucchi A, Ryan D, Konstantakopoulos G, Stroumpa S, Kaçar AS, Renshaw S, et al. Lifetime prevalence of non-suicidal self-injury in patients with eating disorders: a systematic review and meta-analysis. Psychol Med. 2016;46:1345–58.
41. Anestis MD, Silva C, Lavender JM, Crosby RD, Wonderlich SA, Engel SG, et al. Predicting non-suicidal self-injury episodes over a discrete period of time in a sample of women diagnosed with bulimia nervosa: an analysis of self-reported trait and ecological momentary assessment based affective lability and previous suicide attempts. Int J Eat Disord. 2012;45(6):808–11.
42. Claes L, Jiménez-Murcia S, Agüera Z, Castro R, Sánchez I, Menchón JM, et al. Male eating disorder patients with and without non-suicidal self-injury: a comparison of psychopathological and personality features. Eur Eat Disord Rev. 2012;20(4):335–8.
43. Anastasiadou D, Sepulveda AR, Parks M, Cuellar-Flores I, Graell M. The relationship between dysfunctional family patterns and symptom severity among adolescent patients with eating disorders: a gender-specific approach. Women Health. 2016;56(6):695–712.
44. Yen S, Shea MT, Pagano M, Sanislow CA, Grilo CM, McGlashan TH, et al. Axis I and axis II disorders as predictors of prospective suicide attempts: findings from the Collaborative Longitudinal Personality Disorders Study. J Abnorm Psychol. 2003;112(3):375–81.
45. Wang PW, Yen CF. Adolescent substance use behavior and suicidal behavior for boys and girls: a cross-sectional study by latent analysis approach. BMC Psychiatry. 2017;17:392.
46. Carvalho AF, Stubbs B, Vancampfort D, Kloiber S, Maesh M, Firth J, et al. Cannabis use and suicide attempts among 86,254 adolescents aged 12–15 years from 21 low- and middle-income countries. Eur Psychiatry. 2019;56:8–13.
47. Shalit N, Shoval G, Shlosberg D, Feingold D, Lev-Ran S. The association between cannabis use and suicidality among men and women: a population-based longitudinal study. J Affect Disord. 2016;205:216–24.
48. Borges G, Bagge CL, Orozco R. A literature review and meta-analyses of cannabis use and suicidality. J Affect Disord. 2016;195:63–74.
49. Kokkevi A, Richardson C, Olszewski D, Matias J, Monshouwer K, Bjarnason T. Multiple substance use and self-reported suicide attempts by adolescents in 16 European countries. Eur Child Adolesc Psychiatry. 2012;21(8):443–50.

50. Kaley S, Mancino MJ, Messias E. Sadness, suicide, and drug misuse in Arkansas: results from the Youth Risk Behavior Survey 2011. J Ark Med Soc. 2014;110(9):185–6.
51. Peltzer K, Pengpid S. Early substance use initiation and suicide ideation and attempts among school-aged adolescents in four Pacific Island countries in Oceania. Int J Environ Res Public Health. 2015;12:12291–303.
52. DeJong TM, Overholser JC, Stockmeier CA. Apples to oranges? A direct comparison between suicide attempters and suicide completers. J Affect Disord. 2010;124(1–2):90–7.
53. Flensborg-Madsen T, Knop J, Mortensen EL, Becker U, Sher L, Grønbaek M. Alcohol use disorders increase the risk of completed suicide—irrespective of other psychiatric disorders. A longitudinal cohort study. Psychiatry Res. 2009;167(1–2):123–30.
54. O'Boyle M, Brandon EA. Suicide attempts, substance abuse, and personality. J Subst Abuse Treat. 1998;15(4):353–6.
55. Molero Y, Zetterqvist J, Binswanger IA, Hellner C, Larsson H, Fazel S. Medications for alcohol and opioid use disorders and risk of suicidal behavior, accidental overdoses, and crime. Am J Psychiatry. 2018;175(10):970–8.
56. Landi N, Montoya J, Kober H, Rutherford HJ, Mencl WE, Worhunsky PD, et al. Maternal neural responses to infant cries and faces: relationships with substance use. Front Psych. 2011;2:32.
57. Strathearn L. Maternal neglect: oxytocin, dopamine and the neurobiology of attachment. J Neuroendocrinol. 2011;23(11):1054–65.
58. Hans LL, Bernstein VJ, Henson LG. The role of psychopathology in the parenting of drug-dependent women. Dev Psychopathol. 1999;11:957–77.
59. Suchman NE, DeCoste CL, McMahon TJ, Dalton R, Mayes LC, Borelli J. Mothering from the inside out: results of a second randomized clinical trial testing a mentalization-based intervention for mothers in addiction treatment. Dev Psychopathol. 2017;29(2):617–36.
60. James LM, Taylor J. Impulsivity and negative emotionality associated with substance use problems and cluster B personality in college students. Addict Behav. 2007;32(4):714–27.
61. Cohen P, Chen H, Crawford TN, Brook JS, Gordon K. Personality disorders in early adolescence and the development of later substance use disorders in the general population. Drug Alcohol Depend. 2007;88(Suppl 1):S71–84.
62. Roane BM, Taylor DJ. Adolescent insomnia as a risk factor for early adult depression and substance abuse. Sleep. 2008;31(10):1351–6.
63. Wong MM, Brower KJ. The prospective relationship between sleep problems and suicidal behavior in the National Longitudinal Study of Adolescent Health. J Psychiatr Res. 2012;46(7):953–9.
64. McCall WV, Black CG. The link between suicide and insomnia: theoretical mechanisms. Curr Psychiatry Rep. 2013;15(9):389.
65. Winsper C, Tang NKY. Linkages between insomnia and suicidality: prospective associations, high-risk subgroups and possible psychological mechanisms. Int Rev Psychiatry. 2014;26(2):189–204.
66. Chu C, Hom MA, Rogers ML, Stanley IH, Ringer-Moberg FB, Podlogar MC, et al. Insomnia and suicide-related behaviors: a multi-study investigation of thwarted belongingness as a distinct explanatory factor. J Affect Disord. 2017;208:153–62.
67. Singhal A, Ross J, Seminog O, Hawton K, Goldacre MJ. Risk of self-harm and suicide in people with specific psychiatric and physical disorders: comparisons between disorders using English national record linkage. J R Soc Med. 2014;107(5):194–204.
68. Tietjen GE, Brandes JL, Peterlin BL, Eloff A, Dafer RM, Stein MR, et al. Childhood maltreatment and migraine (part II). Emotional abuse as a risk factor for headache chronification. Headache. 2010;50:32–41.
69. Singh S, Taylor C, Kornmehl H, Armstrong AW. Psoriasis and suicidality: a systematic review and meta-analysis. J Am Acad Derm. 2017;77(3):425–40.
70. Roberts E, Wessely S, Chalder T, Chang CK, Hotopf M. Mortality of people with chronic fatigue syndrome: a retrospective cohort study in England and Wales from the South London and Maudsley NHS Foundation Trust Biomedical Research Centre (SLaM BRC) Clinical Record Interactive Search (CRIS) Register. Lancet. 2016;387:1638–43.

71. Smith WR, Noonan C, Buchwald D. Mortality in a cohort of chronically fatigued patients. Psychol Med. 2006;36(9):1301–6.
72. Tietjen GE, Brandes JL, Peterlin BL, Eloff A, Dafer RM, Stein MR, et al. Childhood maltreatment and migraine (part III). Association with comorbid pain conditions. Headache. 2010;50:42–51.
73. Jones GT. Psychosocial vulnerability and early life adversity as risk factors for central sensitivity syndromes. Curr Rheumatol Rev. 2016;12(2):140–53.
74. Sachs-Ericsson N, Cromer K, Hernandez A, Kendall-Tackett K. A review of childhood abuse, health, and pain-related problems: the role of psychiatric disorders and current life stress. J Trauma Dissociation. 2009;10(2):170–88.
75. Bowden MB, Walsh NJ, Jones AJ, Talukder AM, Lawson AG, Kruse EJ. Demographic and clinical factors associated with suicide in gastric cancer in the United States. J Gastrointest Oncol. 2017;8(5):897–901.
76. Rahouma M, Kamel M, Abouarab A, Eldessouki I, Nasar A, Harrison S, et al. Lung cancer patients have the highest malignancy-associated suicide rate in USA: a population-based analysis. Ecancermedicalscience. 2018;12:859.
77. Riem MME, Doedée ENEM, Broekhuizen-Dijksman SC, Beijer E. Attachment and medically unexplained somatic symptoms: the role of mentalization. Psychiatry Res. 2018;268:108–13.
78. Bizzi F, Ensink K, Borelli JL, Mora SC, Cavanna D. Attachment and reflective functioning in children with somatic symptom disorders and disruptive behavior disorders. Eur Child Adolesc Psychiatry. 2019;28(5):705–17.
79. Hudson JI, Arnold LM, Keck PE Jr, Auchenbach MB, Pope HG Jr. Family study of fibromyalgia and affective spectrum disorder. Biol Psychiatry. 2004;56(11):884–91.
80. Shonkoff JP, Garner AS; Committee on Psychosocial Aspects of Child and Family Health; Committee on Early Childhood, Adoption, and Dependent Care; Section on Developmental and Behavioral Pediatrics. The lifelong effects of early childhood adversity and toxic stress. Pediatrics. 2012;129(1):e232–46.
81. Post RM, Altshuler LL, Leverich GS, Frye MA, Suppes T, McElroy SL, et al. Role of childhood adversity in the development of medical co-morbidities associated with bipolar disorder. J Affect Disord. 2013;147:288–94.

Creating Resilient Systems of Care for Youth, Families, and Clinicians

6

Dickon Bevington

Introduction

This chapter will consider principally the wider *social context* of our therapeutic work. Our premise in doing this is that mentalizing is not just a two-person process; it is just as much a social, cultural, and systemic process, extending well beyond individual therapy and out into the social connections not just of the patient but also of the therapist. Hence, this chapter pays only passing attention to the patient and what may be going on in their head and heart. It pays only a little more attention to what passes back and forth between the patient and their therapist. Crucial though that is, it is important to avoid the trap of believing that such obviously *necessary* skills and understandings on the part of a therapist are *sufficient* to bring about change in ways that are truly sustainable. Falling into that trap involves the therapist possibly assuming a risky role of needing to be a kind of "mentalizing ninja," on whose personal skills and innate mentalizing powers alone meaningful change may depend.

Earlier chapters in this book, which describe mentalizing and its development, have linked the development of this capacity not only to the maturing prefrontal cortex but also to the dyadic relationships that unfold between mother and baby, via processes such as marked mirroring. That we learn to mentalize by experiencing what it is to be mentalized by an attachment figure is at the heart of our understanding of this most human of processes [1]. What has perhaps received rather less coverage in the literature to date is the extent to which any mother's capacity to mentalize her baby depends on her own access to other minds (those of partners, parents, friends, and, failing these, professionals) that are available to mentalize her, marking and mirroring the mother in her navigation of the joys and trials of parenthood. By this token, then, mentalizing is, above all, a networked *social capacity*, supported by attachment relationships and brain biology; it is this assumption that

D. Bevington (✉)
Anna Freud National Centre for Children and Families, London, UK
e-mail: Dickon.Bevington@annafreud.org

L. L. Williams, O. Muir (eds.), *Adolescent Suicide and Self-Injury*,
https://doi.org/10.1007/978-3-030-42875-4_6

underpins the rest of this chapter. A legitimate target for any therapy is the question of not only how we enhance the quality of mentalizing relationships around our patients but also their density and distribution. Moreover, this applies as much to those around ourselves as clinicians within the complex networks of care that we inhabit as it does to our patients.

On the basis of this premise about social context, this chapter will discuss the following:

1. Joining existing systems as part of mentalizing
2. A general psychopathology factor (p-factor) and epistemic trust
3. Social connectivity research
4. Addressing disintegration across networks

Part 1: Joining Existing Systems as Part of Mentalizing

Perhaps a common misconception by clinicians is that our work involves the creation of new systems of help around our clients or patients. This is a profoundly "professional-centric" perception and one that very rarely, if ever, accords with the lived experience of those we wish to help. In that sense it represents a profound failure of our mentalizing and a misunderstanding of how the process of help actually works. A more accurate representation is that *we only ever join existing systems of help*—networks of relationships between and around our patients, across which "help" flows in many different forms.

Some of this help may not look at all helpful or safe from a professional perspective. A young person's drug dealer may be about as far from my perception of "help" as they could be, but let's examine this from my patient's perspective. The dealer offers almost complete on-demand availability; what they offer is securely predictable in relation to my patient's expectancies; and in addition to the (albeit teleological) relief from unbearable mental states that their physical product may offer, they may also offer employment opportunities and even security. Of course, many other people in my patient's existing network of help will be much less controversial as "helpers" than a dealer! Family members, faithful friends, or other professionals will—except in the case of the most radically dislocated patients—all have some kind of connection, to a greater or lesser degree. As a therapist, I had better understand the kind of "competition" that I am up against in the race to be helpful to my patient, with a certain amount of humility as to how choices are made regarding whose wares are "bought" in this marketplace of help.

It is almost inevitable in such situations that among this collection of individuals, there will be different ideas and understandings about the nature of the difficulties requiring help, about the kinds of help (or interventions) that are likely to be helpful, and about whose responsibility it should be to deliver such help. One of the most dispiriting features of helping networks is when they seem to fall into operating in ways that replicate this "disintegration."

For now, it is important to be clear that we are all vulnerable to rivalries and to the temptations of positioning ourselves or finding ourselves positioned as the best, the most helpful, or the most important part of any helping network. For instance, as a therapist, my involvement in the life of my patient is likely to be very much more temporary than that of others in their social network. What if my skillful ability to create a deep and trusting relationship with my patient is achieved only at the cost of "showing up" one or more of these other figures? Just as drug treatments are well known to carry with them the risk of unwanted or harmful (iatrogenic) effects, so it is important for the therapist to be alert to that fact that, in the complex arena of help-giving and help-receiving that is mediated by human relationships, there are parallel pitfalls to be avoided.

Part 2: A General Psychopathology Factor and Epistemic Trust

Let us step back a moment to consider our patients' lifetime accumulation of significant psychological suffering; disorders of mental health are balanced against resiliencies. Large and important studies in adult populations [2] and then in adolescent populations [3] have examined the stability across time firstly of *diagnostic categories* and then of *clusters* such as "internalizing" and "externalizing" disorders, with attention focusing on what has been described as a "general psychopathology factor" (*p-factor*) lying behind even these clusters. This number is mathematically determined, with higher numbers indicating a greater psychological burden. What is important to note is that this p-factor is significantly *the most predictive of chronic and severe need, independent of clusters or individual diagnoses.* Patients with a high p-factor are at much higher risk of having more chronic, riskier, and more "treatment-resistant" conditions than those with low p-factors. Even if low-p-factor individuals might initially have had very severe symptoms fitting clear diagnoses, these individuals are statistically still more likely to respond to evidence-based treatments and to recover their function and well-being.

This has inevitably led to debate about precisely what such a p-factor is actually a measure of. At present, perhaps the most compelling explanation [4] is that the p-factor may represent a proxy measure of the extent, or lack, of adaptability in an individual's epistemic trust. As you will recall from Chap. 1, epistemic trust is the ability for individuals to be open, accept, and *use help from another in the face of challenges*. It appears that if they have a high capacity for epistemic trust, even severely affected individuals with a low p-factor may do much better over time than another person with initially less obviously dramatic mental health symptoms.

For people with high p-factors, the "epistemic superhighway" is commonly found to be damaged in two specific ways. First, their capacity for epistemic trust can be sealed over—a condition described as "epistemic hypervigilance." For these individuals, significant paranoia in relation to offers of help (perhaps, in particular, professional help) may be a manifestation of this condition. Second, their epistemic trust system may be wide open such that they appear to trust anyone or everyone, regardless of how unhelpful a person's offers of "help" (those from their drug dealer, for instance) may be.

If, regardless of the specific presenting mental health symptoms or their severity, it is in fact an individual's capacity for adaptive epistemic trust that most determines the depth and extent of their lifetime disability, then this is *highly relevant* to consider when treating patients. Consider that the vast majority of mental health services tend to focus on creating detailed assessments of need and then matching these needs to the best available specialized "delivery mechanisms." While this approach works rather well for patients with low p-factors (those with robust epistemic trust capabilities), it is less successful for those at highest risk, either because they can only engage the system of care thrust upon them with "epistemic hypervigilance" or because they have an inability to discriminate whom to have epistemic trust in.

For this especially vulnerable group, finding ways to build their capacity for adaptive epistemic trust is therefore key. Thus, we urge individual therapists to avoid the urge to become a "mentalizing ninja," as discussed earlier, and instead to pay close attention to the pre-existing networks of help that we join, as therapists, in order to assist in co-constructing a more adaptive capacity for epistemic trust with the young person. Consider the following:

- In their existing network of help, who does the young person currently experience as trustworthy or helpful?
- Who does the young person most experience as "getting" them? (This is a much less technocratic way of describing and identifying the accurate mentalizing of the client by a worker or informal "helper.")
- What might a new worker most usefully learn from these relationships?

Epistemic trust is "won" when a potential helper is perceived as accurately construing the nature and causes of suffering—when the young person perceives that person as showing them that they have a good enough idea of what it is like to be in their shoes. For many young people who function with a closed epistemic highway (hypervigilant), this often means the helper may not actually, at first, be *you* (the therapist) or any expert in mental health.

Coming to trust a potential helper like this is, of course, made easier if the person in front of me looks and sounds as though they have not only academic knowledge and training but also some kind of lived understanding of my world. Where inequalities of class, culture, gender, ethnicity, and power intrude, this is perhaps not inevitably harder, but often is harder. Many therapists, as relatively powerful figures in a network, may thus experience themselves as being at an instant disadvantage in relation to other people in their patients' existing networks of help. Not uncommonly, epistemic trust may be more apparent in the relationship between a young person and a school counselor, favorite teacher, or coach (or yes, even their drug dealer) than in their relationship with their therapist. Remember that for a "professional helper" there is a balance that must be struck between "knowing" (as a qualified expert) and the mentalizing "not-knowing" stance. Let not hubris be the guide when engaging a person with a maladaptive epistemic trust system. Humility, compassion, and humor in the context of genuine curiosity will allow for progress.

Part 3: Social Connectivity Research

Dyads, Triads, Strong and Weak Ties, Structural Holes, Brokerage, and Closure

The *systems of care* referred to in the title of this chapter might give the impression of referring to *managed systems*, with the implication of their being under control and operating in a coordinated way, with clearly defined lines of authority and accountability. As the preceding paragraphs have made clear, whatever local or national organizing principles underlie the provision of health and social care in any setting, the systems of care that we must acknowledge and work within are much better described as *social networks that rely on more opaque influences, shared understandings, and brokerage by third parties.*

Here, alongside psychologists, sociologists, anthropologists, and mathematicians in the field of *social network analysis* (SNA) have introduced frameworks and concepts that offer real promise to the mental health system. A disclaimer is necessary at this point: SNA is a huge field of study, from which only a few key principles are excerpted here; these are presented humbly in the hope that they not only open pathways toward effective action in therapeutic work but also do justice to the deep and complex scholarship upon which they are based. Good introductory texts exist, including Kadushin [5].

First, a few key definitions:

SNA maps Social networks of people, drawn as arrays of nodes and ties.

Nodes Individual people within the network, drawn as dots, circles, squares, etc.

Ties Lines between nodes, representing relationships. Additional qualitative data can be added in the form of thickness/color/texture/arrows, etc., to represent strength or other qualities, though at the risk of flooding the map with too much complexity for the observer to interpret.

Dyad A social network that comprises only two nodes (a couple, or pairing).

Triad A social network with three nodes.

Clique A small network of four or more, in which every node is connected directly to every other node.

Density The measure of how many connections a social network is composed of, in relation to the maximum possible connections between those nodes (which can be expressed numerically as a ratio). For example, if there is a triad, a maximum of three interconnections are possible; with a group of four, there are a total of six possible connections.

Structural hole This is a node that is the sole *bridge* between one subgroup within a network and another. The only way for elements of one subgroup to connect with elements of the other is via the structural hole.

Why might a therapist co-create an SNA map? Experience from the AMBIT (Adaptive Mentalization-Based Integrative Treatment) program (see endnotes and Bevington et al. [6]) suggests that co-creating simple hand-drawn social network maps of the helping figures around a patient offers particular windows or lenses onto these networks that can inform and enrich therapist and patient behaviors. The effort here is to find a way to conceptualize (and then help) the functioning of a distributed network of help without collapsing this into an egocentric or single perspective that denies the many different minds and intentions that are at work. Put more simply, these SNA mapping exercises offer a perspective on mentalizing the network surrounding and involving the young person.

An SNA map becomes *much more* interesting and informative, sometimes revealing otherwise hidden structures and patterns, if the same questions about relationships are asked not just of the patient about each worker they relate to, but also of each worker about the ties they have with all other members of that network—if the map comes to be based upon data rather than just mentalized opinion, as it were. These data-derived SNA maps are what sociologists and mathematicians have studied. If there was an interest in epistemic trust and help across a network, for instance, possible questions *for each member about every other member* might be:

- How much contact do you have with X? (0 = none, 1 = infrequent, 2 = frequent)
- How helpful do you find X? (0 = not at all helpful, 1 = partly helpful, 2 = helpful)
- How much do you feel X understands your situation? (0 = not at all, 1 = partly, 2 = well enough)

The critical point here is that it is not just our patients who are in helping relationships with professional or informal helpers; helpers are helped to greater or lesser degrees by each other, as well, and this is not information that is generally shared explicitly across networks. A therapist and their patient can guess (or try to mentalize) the relationships between other workers, but in much more complex mapping exercises such as this, the use of computer programs is also possible; these create a "model of best fit" based on actual data from survey questions about such relationships. The science of SNA examines the common structures revealed in this way, attempting to relate these to function and outcomes. A landmark description of this approach has been written by Ronald Burt [7].

Triads

With three nodes—a *triad*—complexity begins. In this sense, the triad is described as "the building block of society." The maximum possible density in a triad sees each node connected to both of the others (Figs. 6.1 and 6.2).

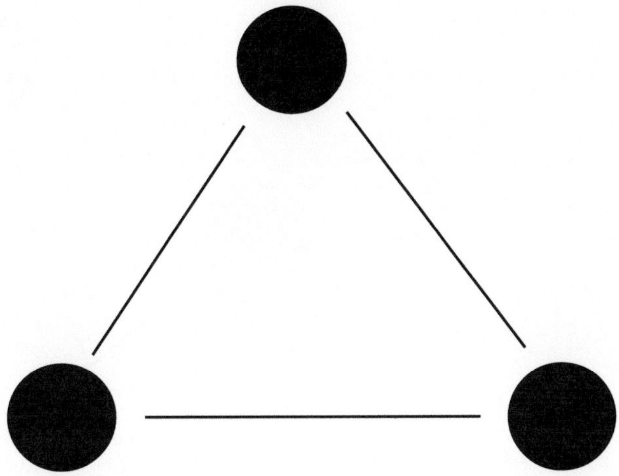

Fig. 6.1 A stable triad: high density

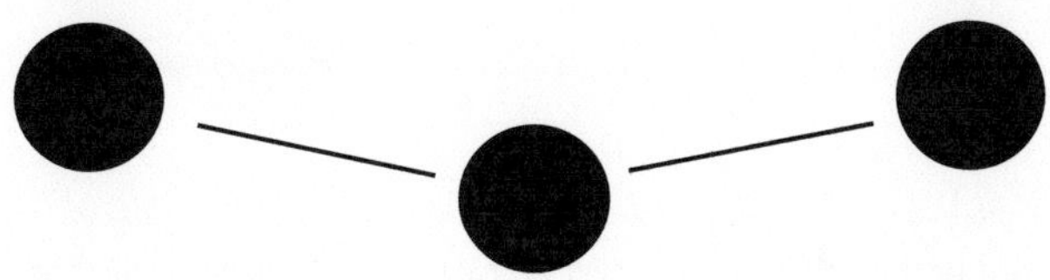

Fig. 6.2 A triad with a broker: low density

A lower-density arrangement would see them arrayed in a line, the central node having ties to both of the others, but those two being *unconnected* to each other. This gives the middle node a certain amount of influence or power, as unless the other two nodes form a direct relationship *independent* of it, it controls their access to each other and holds the potential for creative connectivity. At the same time, a well-intended failure to represent one of the two accurately to the other, or an abuse of that power (for instance, deliberately keeping the other two elements apart as a "divide and rule" strategy or "charging" too much for its role as the "matchmaker") could lead to an unplanned pairing between the other two nodes, uniting in their resistance to the "bad broker," so there is *risk* involved in this position, as well as power. We will return to this ambivalent status in discussing what are referred to rather unpoetically as "structural holes."

When a triad has a density of 1 (ties present between all three nodes), it tends to be a more stable arrangement, regardless of whether all are positive ("My friend's friend is my friend") or whether two are united in mutual resistance to the third ("My enemy's enemy is my friend"). It is reasonable to suggest that mentalizing is promoted in such an arrangement, most simply because the introduction of a third party to a dyad creates the inevitability of another perspective and thereby the possibility for curiosity ("How do you come to see A's behavior like *that*?"). Networks can be analyzed mathematically to ascertain the density not just of ties but also of triads. A higher concentration of triads across a network tends to correlate with greater stability. In considering the network around a patient, it can be helpful to consider how any difficult dyadic relationship in that network might be stabilized by

Fig. 6.3 A clique

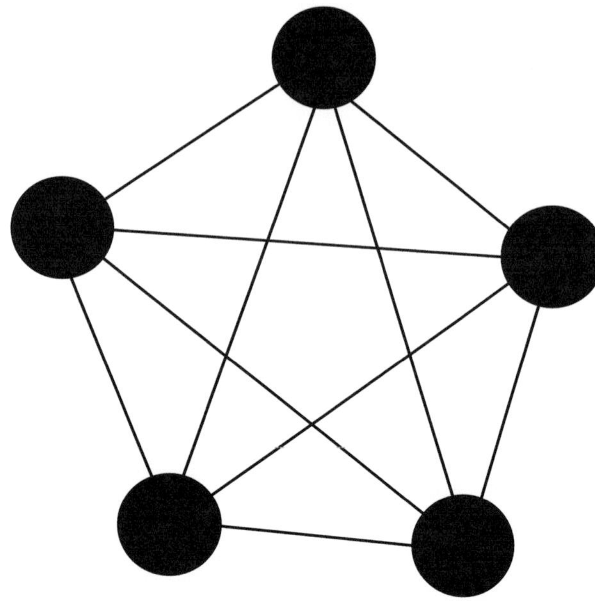

planned efforts to involve that dyad with a helpful third party to create a triad. This has been referred to as "bridging" in systemic practice; the third party will ideally have (or be able to build) relationships of epistemic trust with both parties.

Cliques (Fig. 6.3), as defined above, have four nodes or more, with a high density of strong ties. Such structures tend to be very stable over time, holding each other to strict cultural or practice rules (a good thing in the context of safeguarding and clinical risk) but often at the cost of becoming highly inflexible and perhaps even self-serving and relatively impenetrable by outsiders—and even repressive of their membership. Gangs or extremely isolated families are commonly cited examples, but readers' clinical experience may suggest some small clinical or care teams they have known in practice that have approached this configuration, along with some of these less-helpful behavioral correlates. So, increasing the density of ties across a whole network beyond a certain point does not necessarily increase its functional efficiency; indeed, it is often precisely the *gaps* between clusters that enable these small subgroups to focus on salient information and to process it efficiently where required, while the bridges between them and other parts of the wider network allow efficient transfer and transactions where these matter.

Strong and Weak Ties

This leads us to another area that SNA research has highlighted: the differences between *strong* and *weak ties* (Fig. 6.4). Above, we have mainly addressed strong ties, where there are regular contacts and valued exchanges between nodes. Weak

Fig. 6.4 Strong and weak ties

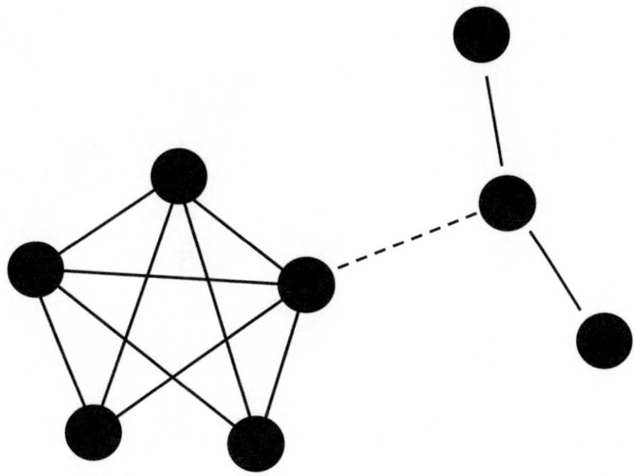

ties are, perhaps paradoxically, at least as important in a network as the strong ones [8], as these are often the ways in which new information (including access to help) flows from greater distances across networks, through which change and difference may be introduced. In contrast, strong ties are what provide security and constancy (with the risk of these working against change where it is required or desired). with a weak tie is often all a therapist has to work with when they first begin to engage with a vulnerable young person and their family, as someone from "another world"; through work on the therapeutic relationship and the creation of security in this relationship, the hope is that it will increase in strength. Equally, as a therapist, I will hope to have strong ties with my team members to provide me with sufficient security to preserve my own mentalizing in situations of anxiety and to hold me to agreed protocols for safety, but it is most commonly weak ties that connect me, as a therapist, to many of the other professionals across a multi agency network. If we work for different agencies, or even just different departments, I may have only passing contact or a "right" to approach these other professionals, simply because of our shared status as workers in allied fields. Attending to the weak ties in a young person's existing network of help may be crucial in developing ideas about how to strengthen its resilience.

Structural Holes

Understanding weak ties, and the idea of how one node might often serve as a "bridge" between two others, leads to another helpful concept from SNA: the notion of "*structural holes*" (Fig. 6.5). A structural hole is the term used to describe a node that is the sole bridge between one subgroup within a network and another. The only way for elements of one subgroup to connect with elements of the other is via the structural hole. Structural holes have rather paradoxical or contradictory qualities. On the one hand, they are imbued with very significant

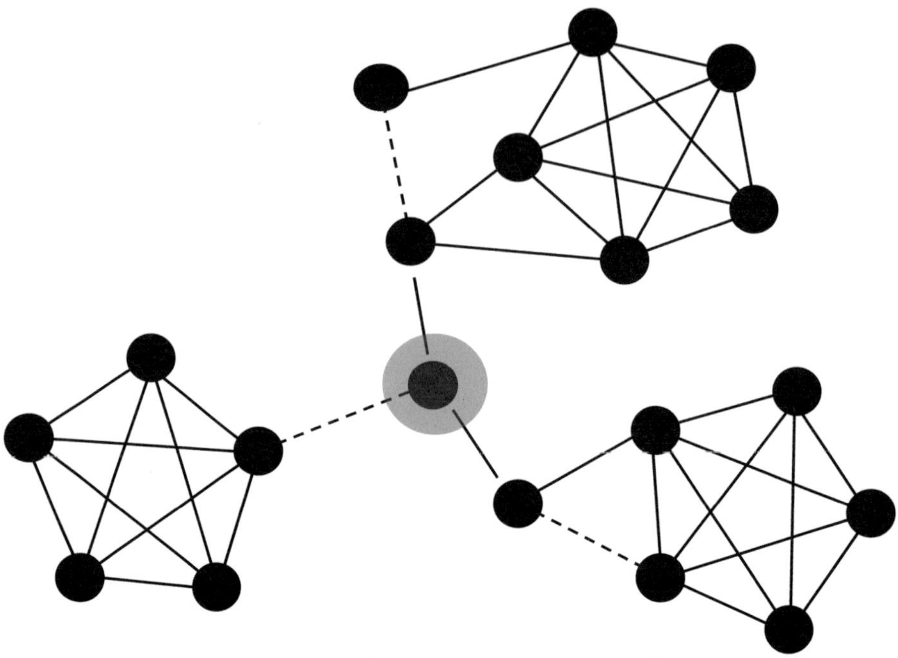

Fig. 6.5 A structural hole

influence or power in a network, as they control access between different parts; they can use this position to adopt a "divide and rule" strategy, controlling how information about different parts of the network is shared, or not. *In an important sense, our patients have this power in the networks of help around them: they are quite frequently the only link between different parts of the wider professional network and are almost always the only path into their own private or informal network of help* (extended family, friends, gang members, etc.). At a more basic level, without our patients, we professionals would have little reason or justification to be in the field at all!

On the other hand, the position of a structural hole is often one of vulnerability and stress: if control and influence depend on a certain amount of keeping people apart, then there are risks attached to those people finding their way into relationships that are not mediated by the structural hole. A simple example of this is a phenomenon that many therapists will recognize, which explains why, as professionals, we are always vulnerable to receiving biased negative feedback about the professional networks within which we must function. On meeting a young person, it is not uncommon to hear accounts of other professionals that are less than flattering: this person was "never available," that one is "only interested in himself," and another "doesn't really listen." It is easy for the therapist hearing these accounts to allow a small flame of competitiveness to take hold; how satisfying it is to be more available and more humbly and empathically engaged than those others! At the same time, a drip feed of these negative connotations about the rest of the professional network easily feeds the kinds of professional mythologies that position me, or my team, as the good outliers in an otherwise broken system, and so the minds and intentions that comprise the other parts of that system are not really investigated or mentalized. Systems are naturally mindless, but they are composed of individual minds. Another risk to the structural hole (here, the patient) is that instead of "buying" the image of fatally flawed professional colleagues, we adopt a judgmental position toward the "ungrateful" or "duplicitous" tale-teller. Of course, there are many reasons why a patient (operating here as a structural hole in the network) might say such things. There are indeed professionals who sometimes function in ways less helpful than they might or should be, but, equally, a patient talking in this way may be communicating as much about what they want me *not* to be (and, by default, offering me advice on how I could behave in order to be more helpful) as they are about the actual people they describe.

Brokerage and Closure

Finally, two other helpful terms for describing these contradictory or balanced forces at work in networks are *brokerage* and *closure*. Brokerage tends to be a function of structural holes (bringing the right people together) and is associated with *effectiveness* in stimulating change—albeit with risks attached, as described above. Closure, on the other hand, relates to the need for systems to provide *safety and control* through the building and maintaining of dense and stable ties (a higher density of triads and strong ties, with less isolated and powerful—yet vulnerable—structural holes or isolated dyads) [7]. At times, one or the other of these forces will be more salient in a particular case, and the challenge for any worker considering the networks around their patient is to find and adjust the balance of these two rather contradictory processes at particular points in time. As the following sections will emphasize, the fragile balancing of often competing or contradictory tasks is at the heart of most therapeutic work, and so an individual therapist rarely, if ever, experiences their work as wholly comfortable. As we know, in conditions of discomfort or uncertainty, our own capacity for mentalizing is challenged.

Part 4: Addressing Disintegration Across Networks

Disintegration Versus Integration

In deciding to help young people who have self-injured or contemplated suicide, it is axiomatic that this work makes therapists anxious. Moreover, we recognize the fact that anxiety in a professional is often closely followed by feelings of professional shame ("I feel anxious, but my colleagues never seem quite as anxious, and that must mean that I am no good at this work.") Shame, in turn, is the enemy of help-seeking behaviors; one hides away in shame rather than going open-handedly to a colleague for help. In training many workers over nearly two decades, we have found it helpful to assert that it is proper, or even essential, that a worker *should* feel anxious (if not all the time, or to extremes). To feel no anxiety in a field where the risks are so many, and the price of failure so high, would indicate a *pretend-mode* functioning that is certainly not mentalizing. So the conundrum is that this work of trying to help our patients to mentalize frequently makes us anxious, which is the enemy of our own mentalizing and of the help-seeking that might restore our mentalizing. In states of non-mentalizing, the therapist is at much higher risk of not only failing to mentalize the patient or their self but also—and perhaps even more easily—failing to mentalize the other parts of the helping network.

Different teams commissioned to address specific kinds of problems often defined by different explanatory frameworks (biological, social–ecological, systemic, psycho analytic, etc.) accordingly emphasize the significance of "their" problems (and the necessity for their leadership) in situations where *co-morbidity* is present, at times with certainty that approaches psychic equivalence. Thus, workers—understandably invested in their specific trainings and roles—unsurprisingly diverge at the level of their *explanations* for a patient's difficulties and around the specific *interventions* that might be indicated. In hard-pressed services where resources are scarce, there is a third level at which frustrated disagreement (which we categorize as a failure to mentalize the other players in the network) can erupt, and that involves who carries *responsibility* for delivering a particular kind of help that is required; this is perhaps more apparent where a system is made up of multi disciplinary teams. These differences may be inconsequential as regards outcomes for our patients, even if they frustrate workers, but there is always a risk that they contribute to or even exacerbate harms, mirroring the fractured and conflicted families that many patients have known. A tool building on these ideas—the *disintegration grid*—is presented below.

It is helpful in this context to apply a *systematic reframing* of professional expectations of complex multi professional networks, one that avoids attributional errors (blaming differences on personal, even moral, failures) and instead *sees disintegration as the natural resting state* of these arrays of human endeavor. Just occasionally, of course, there sadly is cause to call out individual malpractice, but in practice it is very rare that one professional starts their day with the intention of disabling or contradicting the best therapeutic efforts of others; these things just happen *inevitably*. We do better to develop structured ways of predicting, mentalizing, and responding, so as to minimize the harms from these inevitable, though endlessly reconfigured, forms of disintegration.

To do so requires more than one mind because the entropic forces within which we work are too powerful for individual "mentalizing ninjas" to counteract them alone. An essential part of our work, therefore, in addition to the face-to-face encounters of therapy, is attending to the purposeful construction of a "team around the worker"—of social networks that can support our own mentalizing as workers.

Mentalizing Team Tasks

This requires specific attention in two directions:

(a) *Team processes directed at creating well-connected teams. Strong ties* between team members provide the security to keep each other's mentalizing alive in situations that repeatedly challenge this; the aim is a team across which workers are encouraged to seek help from each other and in which a lack of this is challenged. This facilitates and supports the creation of powerful individual therapist–patient relationships by offering a corrective balance to the instability that is implicit in deliberately positioning these individual therapists as powerful (yet vulnerable) *structural holes*.
(b) *Team processes addressing the wider network.* It is crucial to acknowledge the necessity for many minds, skills, and resources, so that the complex and reciprocally synergistic problems that underlie the most challenging mental disorders can adequately be addressed by the different people and different kinds of expertise required. However, this, in turn, necessitates purposeful integrative activities addressing the inevitable and endlessly variable disintegrations that will always be recurring across the essential but usually *weak ties* that characterize the more distant inter professional and informal–family connections across such networks.

Developing Well-Connected Teams

Above, we have seen that the creation of dense and strong ties, through a degree of "closure" across a small team within a larger network, promotes security for its members. "Well-connected" teams mentalize one another more accurately, and this in itself increases the sense of safety for members. In addition, a strong shared team culture supports authentic compliance with safety protocols in ways that top-down managerial dictates alone could never hope to achieve, despite the best intentions of any manager. In order for any strong team culture to be sustained over time (especially in a work environment where the turnover of employees is often high), the presence of social rituals and disciplines protects against improvements in practice becoming diluted or lost.

Well-connected teams value supervisory structures. A mentalizing four-step approach to inter professional help-seeking conversations, called *Thinking Together* [9], emphasizes the importance of mentalizing one's professional colleague when they ask for help, at least as much as mentalizing their patient. The four steps are as follows:

1. *Marking the Task*

   The naming of this step deliberately calls to mind "marked mirroring." Here, the thrust is to "kick-start" the mentalizing of the help-seeker, insisting that they "start as we mean to continue" in *efforts to mentalize*. It is about creating clear boundaries around a conversation that can occur in a variety of settings. It will include an explicit allocation of available time for this to take place.

The help-giver will not proceed further into conversation until they are as clear as they can be about *what kind of help is being sought by this colleague of theirs*. This requires some reciprocal effort to define what a helpful end point of the conversation would look like ("What is the intention underlying your opening of this conversation?" or "What would it look or feel like if I were successful in helping you in the way I assume you hope I will?"). It requires the help-seeker, in a modest way, first to stop and mentalize their *own* behavior in turning to their colleague for help. It helps to ground the conversation in the emotional here and now.

Commonly, without an explicit team culture that expects this discipline, help-seeking conversations miss this step out and begin with the help-seeker giving (or pouring out) an account of their problem. This creates a dual task for the helper: first to try to guess what the help-seeker actually wants ("What is the task for me here?") and second to follow what it is that their help-seeking colleague is saying, so as to understand their state of mind and the scenario in question. In conditions of stress, this may limit the capacity of the helper either to listen accurately to the story when it does come or to frame their response in ways that are contingent upon the help-seeker's felt need. In these circumstances, it is often easier to respond with cleverness (pretend mode) or mechanistically (teleologically) than it is to address what a colleague actually needs.

Examples of the kinds of task that a help-seeker may "mark" for a colleague are extremely diverse: "I want a couple of new ideas of what to do next because I feel my patient is disengaging," "I want to know if my risk plan makes sense," "I want to stop feeling angry toward my patient," "I want to make sense of why the social worker is behaving like this," etc.

Teams should work to create a culture that explicitly acknowledges the inevitability of occasionally being overwhelmed and the expectation of help-seeking as a behavioral norm, so that marking such tasks to each other becomes ordinary, not an exception.

2. *Stating the Case*

   Here, the help-seeker is given some time to share the relevant "bones" of the story that their colleague might need in order to help them with the task. Again, there is a toughness in this step: both parties have explicitly "contracted in" for a Thinking Together exchange, and this gives the help-giver permission to exert a certain amount of control, ensuring (with the agreed time limits in mind) that the help-seeker does not slip into exhaustive over inclusivity and "storytelling," which is a common (pretend mode and teleological) response to the anxiety implicit in our work. ("If only I can include every detail, things will be clear.")

3. *Mentalizing the Moment*

   Here, there is a deliberate (marked, as it were) change of gear, as if temporarily the boundaries of the conversation were relaxed, and minds are allowed to "play" with what has gone before. Again, without having Thinking Together as an explicit social discipline, this step is commonly overlooked in helping conversations: we often move directly from a telling of the problem to a telling of the solution. Crucially, this step is where the spotlight initially turns onto the help-*giver* in the pairing: the help-seeker is invited to sit back momentarily. As for the help-giver, the first person they are invited to mentalize as accurately as possible at this point is *not* the patient or other players in the case presented, but *the colleague in front of them.* The logic behind this is that under conditions of stress, errors in mentalizing are liable to arise. Almost by definition, it is assumed that it is some stress that has driven their help-seeking colleague to initiate this dialogue. We know that the most powerful way to restore a person's mentalizing is for them to have the experience of being accurately mentalized by a trusted other, and that these are the preconditions for epistemic trust [10].

4. *Return to Purpose*

   These conversations are task focused and are designed to be carried out in busy work settings, so it is the responsibility of the help-giver to help steer the conversation into its closing phase. Now the help-seeker is invited to reflect on whether, in the light of the preceding exchanges, any solutions have arisen in their own mind. The help-giver may offer their own reflections and, if necessary, suggestions too, always bearing in mind the originally defined task: the purpose of these conversations is to offer contingent care for the help-seeking colleague to address *their* need (rather than to offer help-givers an opportunity to exert power or demonstrate prowess!). Clearly, this is also a place for risks that may have gone unacknowledged to be explored and responded to. However, the overarching intention behind this structured approach is to *help restore a colleague's mentalizing*. Thinking together is, of course, the most ordinary of interactions (one colleague asking another for help). By focusing attention on doing this in more systematic ways, the intention is to contribute to the efficient functioning of the team by developing and sustaining an explicit team culture that places as much value on mentalizing the minds of team members as it does on mentalizing the minds of patients. The very fact of creating these four steps as a shared social discipline can act as an explicit marker of team culture.

There can be a direct impact on patients cared for under this approach, too. Therapists who make reference to the help they get from colleagues in relation to their work, naming these helpers and describing the ways in which they have been helped by them (to understand something differently, to get access to a resource, etc.), *are using their own relationship of epistemic trust with their patient to model and normalize the process of help-seeking*. What is on show to the young person is the notion of a necessary "back-up team." As the young person observes this, the invitation is for them to consider how their own back up team looks at this point in time, and whether there may be ways to strengthen ties, or find new ones, so that it could function in similar ways. Finally, as a means of supporting the referral of an epistemically hypervigilant youth to a more specialized colleague, it is often much more effective for a professional who has created some epistemic trust with them to speak *not* of "how good that person will be for you!" but instead to speak of "how helpful that person has been to *me*."

Team Processes Addressing Disintegration in the Wider Network

Disintegration can certainly occur across the strong ties that exist in teams or families, and where it does, it is obviously particularly important to address it. On the other hand, it is usually much easier to spot (or harder to ignore) in such settings. Here, we are more focused on identifying and addressing it when it occurs beyond these immediate relationships and across what we know are the *crucial weak ties of a wider network of help*.

At this juncture, consider using the SNA connectivity maps discussed earlier—produced collaboratively with the young person, using a large sheet of chart paper. Starting with the young person in the middle, all of their most relevant sources of help (formal, informal, conventional, and non-conventional) can be added, with the distances and different line styles/thicknesses between the "players" being used to enrich the information being encoded. In this way, these simple sketches can indicate the extent to which different players are *perceived* (note that these maps are not data driven, as true SNA maps are) to have contact or not, to understand or to help the young person, or to agree with each other or not, etc. As an early means of engaging—and of asserting the humble truth that, as a therapist, I only join *existing* networks of help, rather than creating a brand new one—they have been found to be helpful and acceptable to young people.

A technique for identifying the most salient disintegrations across a network, which offers a more systematic approach to mentalizing its key players, is the *disintegration grid.* A grid is drawn up with *three rows* and then *a column for each of the key players* identified in the given network. The rows are labeled thus:

1. *Explanation* ("What's the problem?")
2. *Intervention* ("What to do?")
3. *Responsibility* ("Who does what?")

The therapist then mentalizes each "player" to consider the most likely "bullet points" that *this person would want to see represented* in relation to the case, at each level. In recording these points, the instruction is always to try to write points that, if they were seen by the player themselves, "would elicit an approving nod." This is, of course, harder than it first appears! The resulting grid will almost inevitably and unsurprisingly reveal a range of different perspectives (along with a number of question marks that may reveal telling areas of ignorance), and most of these differences may have only a marginal impact on network functioning. It will often reveal a smaller number of key points of difference (or conflict) that are unhelpful to the functioning of the whole network, especially in respect of the shared intention (we hope): that the whole network should be helpful to our patient's safety and progress. It is helpful first just to identify at which level the disintegration is occurring: is it at the level of explanations, or interventions, or responsibilities?

In a large network it is rarely feasible to hope to get everyone in the same room, certainly at short notice, although multi professional case conferences themselves are often highly effective ways to reduce the negative impacts of disintegration. Disintegration grids can be extremely helpful ways of notating such multi professional meetings when they do occur. An attending team member can set about recording the different players' comments verbatim in the various cells of the grid as they talk, rather than relying on their own, less reliable, private mentalizing. In the author's experience, multi agency meetings often become curious if this technique is used transparently in such settings but without seeking to impose it upon the group. In turn, this curiosity has often led to the grid being completed collaboratively by the whole group, ideally using a white board. Where this has occurred, it has helped reaffirm the underlying shared intentions in the room (to help the patient) and rekindle curiosity (as good a proxy for "mentalizing" as any) about each other's work, let alone highlighting possible "connecting conversations" that, if facilitated, might reduce or repair a particularly egregious aspect of disintegration.

In the absence of a multi professional meeting, for a therapist who has a limited amount of time per case (especially as regards attending specifically to *network* issues around a case), a grid completed in private or with a colleague can help them focus on where and how to spend a limited amount of "networking time" most efficiently in the coming week. Conducting "connecting conversations" across particular disintegrations sounds simple enough but is, of course, anything but. Here, strategic thinking will be required, and SNA can offer some clues about ways forward. Who are the most helpful other people in this network, who might act as a trusted bridge, or create triads, with the conflicted dyad? Are there already shared weak ties between these two network members that could be strengthened? Where and how does power flow across this dyad, and how might understanding this affect or shape any intervention? Application of theory and practice drawn from mentalizing is, of course, just as relevant in these situations as in any face-to-face therapeutic work; if I wish to get the attention of a professional colleague, and earn some epistemic trust, I had better find ways to accurately mentalize *their* predicament before I issue advice or commands.

Conclusion

Nothing is new; the poet John Donne (1572–1631) wrote:

> *No man is an island entire of itself; every man*
> *Is a piece of the continent, a part of the main.*

This applies to our patients (any patients, but perhaps *especially* young people, who tend to be so much more densely networked than adults), but it also applies to their parents and carers, and to ourselves as their mental health team members. Attention to only one mind, if it is to the exclusion of others on that "main," is unlikely to provide for sustainable change.

Furthermore, any therapeutic work needs to acknowledge that the hours a young person spends in therapy are as a speck in comparison with the other hours spent amid the wider, fragile, and occasionally very risky "networks of help" that we all surround ourselves with. If epistemic trust does its job, it allows for new ideas about how to react, or be, to be taken in by our patients and tried out *beyond* the consulting room—amid these networked interactions. Out there, as therapists, it can feel as though we are limited to simply holding our breath and crossing our fingers, in the hope that the world will be just benign enough first to notice a courageous change in our patient's behavior and then to acknowledge and thereby reinforce it. We are not powerless, however. Apportioning some of our energies and time to building and shaping more effective, more mentalizing networks is possible. Moreover, evidence suggests this need not be done entirely blindly, nor is it entirely in vain.

Key Points

1. Mentalizing is helpfully thought of as a social capacity, not just an individual (prefrontal) capability.
2. The therapist should attend to the existing helping network around the patient, which they join; they are never creating a new network.
3. Epistemic trust does not follow rank, experience, or formal authority, but understanding its presence or absence for a patient is crucial.
4. Understanding (and balancing) the contradictory and ambiguous forces of brokerage and closure across a helping network helps to organize network interventions.
5. Disintegration across complex helping systems is their natural resting state and is only rarely due to malign intent; having systematic approaches to address this is an essential part of any therapeutic work.

For those interested to learn more about employing a mentalizing scaffold to develop systems of care, the author points the reader to AMBIT (Adaptive Mentalization-Based Integrative Treatment) [5]. Most of this chapter is based on the work of the AMBIT program, developed through collaboration between academics and clinicians at the Anna Freud National Centre for Children and Families (London, UK) and multiple local teams located in the UK and internationally. AMBIT is an *open-source* mentalization-based program—partly a therapeutic method (for high-risk, high-complexity, and low-help-seeking populations) and partly a quality improvement approach. It joins with local systems and cultures, encourages local adaptions to support local systems and fit local cultural conditions, and offers a principled stance and a range of core team disciplines. Readers are encouraged to visit the free wiki-manual website: https://manuals.annafreud.org/ambit.

References

1. Fonagy P, Target M. Playing with reality: I. Theory of mind and the normal development of psychic reality. Int J Psychoanal. 1996;77:217–33.
2. Caspi A, et al. The p-factor: one general psychopathology factor in the structure of psychiatric disorders? Clin Psychol Sci. 2014;2(2):119–37.
3. Patalay P, Fonagy P, et al. A general psychopathology factor in early adolescence. Br J Psychiatry. 2015;207(1):15–22.

4. Fonagy P, Luyten P, Campbell C, Allison L. Epistemic trust, psychopathology and the great psychotherapy debate. Society for the Advancement of Psychotherapy. http://www.societyforpsychotherapy.org/epistemic-trust-psychopathology-and-the-great-psychotherapy-debate. Accessed 21 Jul 2019.
5. Kadushin C. Understanding social networks: theories, concepts, and findings. Oxford: Oxford University Press; 2012.
6. Bevington D, Fuggle P, Cracknell L, Fonagy P. Adaptive mentalization-based integrative treatment: a guide for teams to develop systems of care. Oxford: Oxford University Press; 2017.
7. Burt R. Structural holes versus network closure as social capital. In: Lin N, Cook K, Burt R, editors. Social capital: theory and research. Oxford: Transaction; 2001.
8. Granovetter M. The strength of weak ties. Am J Sociol. 1973;78(6):1360–80.
9. Bevington D, Fuggle P, Fonagy P. Applying attachment theory to effective practice with hard-to-reach youth: the AMBIT approach. Attach Hum Dev. 2015;17(2):157–74. https://doi.org/10.1080/14616734.2015.1006385.
10. Fonagy P, Allison E. The role of mentalizing and epistemic trust in the therapeutic relationship. Psychotherapy. 2014;51(3):372–80. https://doi.org/10.1037/a0036505.

Mentalization-Based Treatment Plays Well with Others

7

Carlene MacMillan

Introduction

Over the past decade, a number of different approaches to the treatment of self-harm and suicide have gained traction. Which therapy to choose likely feels confusing not just to clinicians but also to families desperately searching for help. We would argue that no matter which therapeutic approach is chosen, mentalization will have a key role to play if the therapy is to be as effective as possible. From the earlier chapters in this book, you have hopefully gleaned three key principles: mentalizing is a skill we all possess: mentalizing normally goes on and offline for everyone, including the therapist, but especially for patients who may be struggling with suicide or self-injurious thoughts and behaviors; and mentalizing, as a skill set, is important to keep track of for both the patient and the therapist. As we will see below, these principles hold true across a wide range of therapeutic approaches.

The idea that we really should try to "keep the mind in mind" sounds so simplistic that seasoned therapists will sometimes ask if there is anything new to be learned by deliberately incorporating this concept into their work. Even the pioneers of mentalization-based treatment (MBT) have, at times, posed the question of whether MBT is simply "old wine in new bottles" [1] or whether, on the contrary, it offers something genuinely innovative to therapists. They described it at one point as "the least novel therapeutic approach imaginable, simply because it revolves around a fundamental human capacity—indeed, the capacity that makes us human" [2].

Our interpretation, however, is that what the pioneers of MBT accomplished was to bring together biology, attachment research, neuroimaging, and developmental psychology to carefully consider what makes therapy work. Think about this for a minute: why would one human being decide to listen to another human being, especially one they didn't know very well, about their tender internal emotional states?

C. MacMillan (✉)
Brooklyn Minds Psychiatry, Brooklyn, NY, USA
e-mail: carlene.macmillan@brooklynminds.com

L. L. Williams, O. Muir (eds.), *Adolescent Suicide and Self-Injury*,
https://doi.org/10.1007/978-3-030-42875-4_7

Although it may not be exclusively human to decide to place our trust in another [every day, we are learning more about the other creatures we inhabit this planet with], it is, in our humble opinion, FOUNDATIONAL to psychotherapy working [3]. In practice, we posit that this universality means that MBT principles and techniques can be used synergistically with many other schools of therapeutic thought. This can be said for first-wave therapies such as psychoanalysis, second-wave therapies such as cognitive behavioral therapy (CBT), and, finally, to third-wave therapies such as dialectical behavior therapy (DBT) or acceptance and commitment therapy.

If your mental radar is tuned to track how much mentalization is happening for you and the patient in any sort of therapy session, you are off to a good start. Think of mentalization as the therapy equivalent of a high-speed internet connection; you cannot stream the latest episode of your favorite show unless your internet connection is on point, and you cannot effectively generate insight or teach skills unless mentalizing is online. In observing any effective and engaged therapy session, you are likely going to notice that mentalization is happening between the therapist and patient regardless of what primary style of therapy is being offered. In contrast, therapy sessions that are not going so well—remaining superficial or exploding into utter chaos, with slamming doors and tears—feature a much higher percentage of non-mentalized moments, often on the part of both the therapist and the patient (Fig. 7.1).

The three pre-mentalizing modes—pretend mode, psychic equivalence, and teleological mode—can arise in all forms of therapy. So we remind you, dear reader, about the first rule of mentalizing therapy: check for mentalizing. What is the second rule of mentalizing therapy? Get mentalizing back online. Why do we do this? To return to the epistemic trust super highway. Why do we want to be on that highway? To get the patient where they are going as efficiently as possible. From that

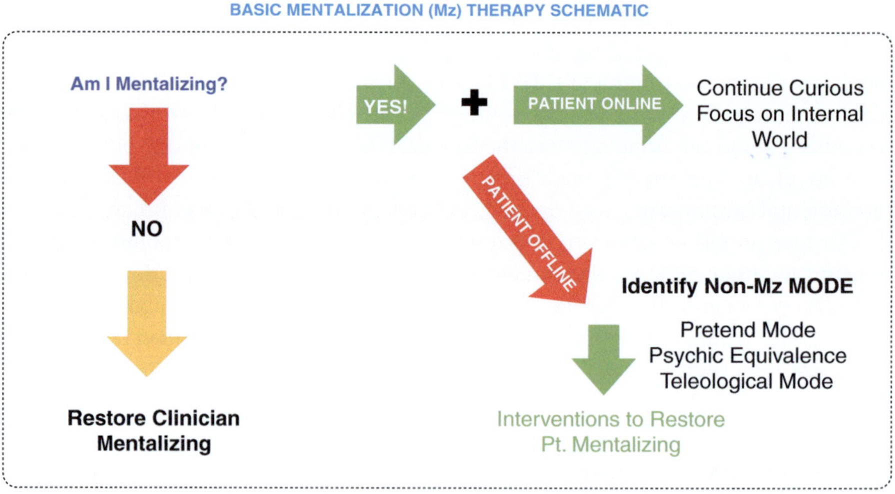

Fig. 7.1 Basic mentalization. *Pt* patient

perspective, mentalizing therapists are wildly accepting of any and all modalities of psychotherapy—first, because we know there is an evidence base showing that a variety of psychotherapies can be effective [4]; and second (and in our minds, more importantly), because we know that not every patient will respond to only one type of therapy. If the evidence pointed to one psychotherapy being the "winner," this book would frankly be unnecessary and you would rightly want your money back. In actuality, the evidence primarily points in the direction of all psychotherapies, if patients actually attend sessions, being only modestly effective. So we see there is still much work to be done for therapy to become even more effective. Finally, there is an open secret in the field of psychotherapy research that points to two additional important facts that should bolster your desire to learn and implement mentalizing theory and skills: first, patients with less severe symptoms generally get better faster and in a more sustained manner than more impaired patients; and second, patients who form a good working alliance (think attachment and epistemic trust) with their therapist tend to get better faster and in a more sustained manner. Finally, an even sneakier secret is that the mentalizing skills of the therapist have a great deal to do with the eventual success (or not) of the therapy, regardless of age, race, gender, years of experience, or therapeutic modality.

Therefore, the primary goal of this chapter is not to convince you, dear reader, to pick MBT over other forms of treatment. Indeed, our team would feel somewhat bereft if you came to such a conclusion. Instead, the goal is to provide evidence of how MBT can be integrated into therapeutic work regardless of the therapy approach. If you feel most comfortable with a dynamic approach, fantastic! Want to do thought charts all day long? Wonderful! Radically accepting a feeling state? Bring it on!

This chapter will discuss the following:

1. How does pretend mode uniquely interfere with psychodynamic therapy, CBT, and DBT?
2. How does psychic equivalence mode uniquely interfere with psychodynamic therapy, CBT, and DBT?
3. How does teleological mode uniquely interfere with psychodynamic therapy, CBT, and DBT?

Pretend Mode

First, let's consider pretend mode. Pretend mode is associated with having too low an affective temperature in the session. A psychodynamic therapist might notice the frequent use of defense mechanisms such as intellectualization, whereas a DBT therapist might say the patient was spending much of the session in "Rational Mind" with very little authentic emotion being let in. It is our job as therapists in these moments to use mentalization techniques to turn up that affective temperature into a range where work can be done.

Most therapists can probably think of sessions where they noticed their own minds were wandering toward what to eat for dinner or feeling frankly bored as the person sitting across from them rambled on, using all sorts of jargon. Talk of various defense mechanisms and how they arose may have been rampant, yet the sessions felt empty and rote. In psychodynamic therapy, this can happen when a patient has "been in therapy since preschool" with little to show for it. The patient has a canned narrative picked up along the way of why they are the way they are, and such articulated insights are ostensibly the goal. The therapist may provide some new and seemingly brilliant interpretations that the patient then incorporates into this non-mentalized pretend mode narrative. This can be very seductive, as it usually feels good when a patient tells a therapist how brilliant they are. For a psychodynamic therapist who has their pretend mode radar on high alert, however, these type of mechanical interactions and feelings of boredom should set off alarm bells. Merely noticing pretend mode does not eradicate it, but it is the first step.

When pretend mode is dominating the session, the therapist can then use MBT techniques such as the use of an unexpected challenge to raise the emotional temperature back to levels where some therapeutic work can get done. Challenges can be pretty random and irreverent. One therapist we know stood up on a table when bored in a session with a jaded teen and shouted, "Cowabunga!" This was not at all what the teen expected, and pretend mode ceased. Using the polarities, we can challenge the patient to move from "self versus other" to get some reflective functioning going. For example, if the patient is focusing on themselves almost exclusively, the therapist can begin asking questions to shift toward thinking about the perspective of others. To really raise the affective temperature, asking the patient to think about the therapist's perspective and what they might be thinking and feeling can suddenly interject the "here and now" into the room. This is, after all, psychodynamic therapy, and generating movement along the MBT polarities is a truly dynamic, lively process. We encourage you to make some waves when the sea is too calm, so to speak. After using your "MBT ninja" skills, you should find yourself on the edge of your seat again, no longer wondering what to eat for dinner. While MBT is designed to encourage reflective functioning rather than generate insights, once reflective functioning is happening, it is almost magical how insights can work their way into sessions in an authentic and connected way.

Pretend mode can also work its way into sessions that focus on more skills-based behavioral therapies such as CBT and DBT. We are thinking here of young people who could teach a class on cognitive distortions or distress tolerance skills, yet they cannot seem to actually use the skills in "real life" in any consistent way. They may be quick to dismiss these treatments as not helpful. So what went wrong? Do they just need to do another round of skills training until it sinks in? Not quite. We would argue that the degree to which the skills were truly internalized and consistently generalized has to do with how mentalized these skills training sessions and coaching calls were. In our practice, our psychologists who would identify as "hard-core behaviorists" have embraced techniques from MBT to make their sessions—well—more hard-core. Let's see how MBT can pair with DBT to get this difficult job done.

First, let's see when our non-mentalized radar should go off during a skills-based therapy session. When an adolescent states that "DBT did not help," it is important to probe to see how the prior therapist connected with them, how lively the sessions were, and whether it seemed like a "real" relationship where one could feel free to be honest. Often when DBT or CBT has not been effective, a young person will state that they filled out diary cards or other worksheets and did homework so as to not "get in trouble," but not in any real sort of way, and that the therapist seemed to be following a protocol but did not seem particularly curious about their perspectives. As Chap. 6 in this book tells us, though, we are wise to not completely pride ourselves on skills the previous therapist reportedly lacked. We know that for mentalizing ninjas, it is important to challenge these blanket statements, much as a great CBT or DBT therapist would. Probe the depth; maybe it is true that DBT did not help, but it is better to more fully dissect these statements in order to avoid similar non-mentalizing encounters. Skills-based therapies are typically more focused on the here and now than traditional psychodynamic therapies, mapping nicely onto MBT's "here and now with us, not then and there with them" philosophy. So if a skills-based session starts to look more like going through the motions than hard work, bringing up what is going on in the room between you and the patient can be revitalizing. This is what we refer to as affect focus or mentalizing the relationship. Saying things like "I wonder if when I assign you therapy homework, you just say you will do it to please me but have no intention to; I would much prefer you to tell me you think it is kind of stupid than pretend and not help you feel better" can deepen the conversation considerably. Not only that, but it can also lead to adjustments being made to the type of assignments so they are things the young person finds genuinely useful. Wouldn't that be transformational therapy helping!

One example of a DBT assignment that can be enhanced by techniques from mentalization is the completion of a chain analysis about the events, thoughts, and feelings that led to a target behavior, such as self-harm, taking place. Embarking on a mentalized chain analysis would involve a conscious effort for the therapist to take a "not-knowing" and curious stance about the thoughts and feelings that come up along the chain, rather than suggest thoughts and feelings that the patient is likely to agree to in an effort to appear agreeable and move the task along. If your patient is stuck and uses the dreaded "J word"—"I don't know, it *just* happened"—you could say, "If I were you in that circumstance, I might have felt really angry. Were you feeling that or not quite?" This is a more subtle not-knowing stance than something that is validating but more certain, such as "Wow, you must have felt angry then!" The former phrasing is more likely to generate a discussion, whereas the latter is likely to generate unexamined agreement. It models that everyone can have a different perspective of the same situation, and we should not assume we know how someone feels; these are tenets of mentalization.

DBT therapists are encouraged to incorporate playful irreverence into their work, and an MBT therapist might say that well-timed irreverence can serve as an effective challenge—a therapeutic maneuver designed to jolt mentalization back online. When working on a chain analysis, a therapist who finds it is getting a bit stale may throw in an unexpected statement such as "and then you pulled out your magic wand and cast a spell to cast out the urges to self-injure, right?" These challenge maneuvers can sometimes fall flat or even offend, but, if done thoughtfully, can often bring a session back to life for the better. While the goal of the DBT therapist conducting the chain analysis may primarily be to introduce points where skills could have been used to prevent a target behavior such as self-injury, the MBT-informed therapist is also keenly interested in looking for the moments where mentalization went offline, understanding that a target behavior such as self-injury is frequently the end result of someone stopping mentalizing at one point due to intense emotions—especially negative feelings about a social encounter—getting in the way. You can use the "rewind" technique to backtrack as far back as the person can remember before things really went off the rails. You can also keep in mind that in doing a chain analysis, once a person has stopped mentalizing, their accounts of subsequent thoughts and feelings that came along the way to the target behavior may be pure conjecture at best. When a young person says, "and then it just happened; I ended up cutting," they may indeed be telling the truth as they recall it, and further attempts to get them to fill out a form with thoughts and feelings may result in pretend mode responses. Instead of hitting a dead end, the DBT therapist would likely gain more traction if they said, "OK, so let's work on what skills you could use next time so as to not get to the point where you are not mentalizing anymore or so you can recognize that you are not and get yourself back on track" than if they focused very much on the moments right before the target behavior. In this framework, one could actually reconceptualize the target behavior that needs work as the collapse of the ability to mentalize into a non-mentalized mode. The typical target behaviors such as self-injury or a suicidal gesture are really more smoke signals that there is a fire of non-mentalized thought happening. In this, a mentalizing therapist is less concerned about the final act than about how to assist the person to stay engaged in mentalizing.

Psychic Equivalence

The pre-mentalizing mode known as psychic equivalence, where feelings equal facts, can also be found across therapy modalities. Unlike pretend mode, which usually accompanies a low affective temperature, psychic equivalence usually shows up on the scene when emotions are too intense and overwhelming.

In insight-oriented psychodynamic therapy, this can take the form of a patient dramatically unraveling in the face of uncertainty in the presence of a therapist who is employing a more reserved stance. The patient may begin to believe all sorts of things, such as that they know the therapist must hate them and think they are evil, despite the absence of any facts suggesting that. The term "borderline" to describe these individuals came about historically in the psychoanalytic literature to convey that in this therapy, the individual could present as being on the border between psychosis and neurosis. We would say the person was in psychic equivalence during these sessions. These harrowing sessions led to the pervasive belief that individuals with borderline personality styles should not be in this type of therapy. However, it is not quite that simple. If a therapist in a session headed in this direction can recognize the signs of psychic equivalence, they can essentially hit the pause button and interject with statements that are curious and validating, if the client can handle that.

If not, they can hit the pause button and switch gears to a completely different, less psychically loaded topic, potentially returning later to the topic that led to the unraveling, if it feels appropriate. This could be later in that session or it could be much later, especially if the topic involves unprocessed trauma. The appearance of psychic equivalence in a psychodynamic session does not mean that this form of therapy is not appropriate; rather, it means that for this individual, it will take a concerted effort to keep the affective temperature from soaring through the roof. The pot of gold at the end of the psychodynamic rainbow here is the eventual development of a trusting, safe holding environment where, eventually, previously triggering topics can be talked about without a collapse of mentalization.

In behavioral therapies such as CBT, psychic equivalence is often front and center as the target of interventions, though that terminology is likely not used. Indeed, in describing MBT to fellow therapists, a description such as "It helps people think more flexibly about different possibilities" can lead to questions about whether or not MBT is any different from CBT. It seems that psychic equivalence is targeted head on by CBT techniques designed to address cognitive distortions. CBT places a heavy emphasis on explicit, controlled mentalizing for individuals who tend to overly rely on automatic, negative implicit ways of thinking about themselves and the world. A behavioral therapist designs exposure hierarchies to help individuals face their implicit and non-mentalized counterproductive and entrenched beliefs. Throughout the process, the therapist asks for ratings of subjective units of distress (SUDS). These ratings are a quantitative metric of what we talk about in MBT as the affective temperature. If the therapist designs an intervention that is too intense, the SUDS score will be too high—mentalization will go offline and no learning of a new outlook will take place. Fear will dominate and reinforce psychic equivalence. If the intervention is not intense enough, the SUDS score will be too low and pretend mode will dominate. Cognitive distortions and obsessive thinking are both attempts by the mind to eradicate uncertainty and simplify the world. Unfortunately, when feelings rather than facts drive this type of thinking, people end up with maladaptive ways to navigate the world. CBT and exposure–response prevention techniques all aim to inject uncertainty into the mix and help the individual build up a tolerance for that unsettling feeling. While CBT has its own lexicon of terms such as catastrophizing or personalization, these are all, at their core, psychic equivalence. MBT's prediction that validation of the feelings behind the distortions, followed by curious exploration (which in CBT can be facilitated with things like thought record CBT worksheets) will lead to more flexible thinking makes sense when seen through this lens. For example, if someone is stuck in thinking they should have done something different and are a total loser, doomed to nothing but future failures, one common CBT technique is to try and imagine what they might say to a friend in a similar situation. This is using the "self versus other" polarity we talk about in MBT to facilitate a move away from the negative and certain way they focus on themselves, to consider an alternative perspective about how they would view the same situation if a friend was in it, and then to apply that perspective back to themselves. This is an active process, and when it goes well, the CBT therapist and patient are both able to mentalize and move past the impasse.

We should also note that over the past several years, a number of computer programs and smartphone apps have been created to deliver CBT in the absence of a therapist. While there are many people who can and do benefit from that approach, for adolescents struggling with very intense emotions that can lead to suicidal thinking or self-injury, having a CBT therapist who is aware of the principles of mentalization can build trust and navigate the affective temperature of a session in ways that a computer program cannot. Machine learning is just not there yet, so no, you are not out of a job! That is not to say these electronic tools have no place in a therapist's toolkit; rather, they may not be sufficient for clients who are prone to rapid descent into pre-mentalized modes when faced with challenges.

Teleological Mode

The final pre-mentalized mode we will explore in the context of non-MBT therapy modalities is teleological mode, also known as "prove-it" or "show-me" mode, where there is a heavy emphasis on actions (or inactions) and certainty around what these actions are intended to mean. More psychodynamically oriented therapists may recognize teleological mode when there are bids for boundary crossings or enactments taking place that feel counterproductive. More cognitive behavioral–oriented therapists, including DBT therapists, may recognize this mode when so-called "treatment interfering" behaviors start taking place or when demands for the therapist's time to provide skills coaching outside sessions ramp up and start to feel like the person is not really asking for skills; rather, they are seeking some intangible connection with the person on the other end of the phone. This is the mode that can be treatment destroying and can lead to some legitimately scary and risky behavior when not noticed and addressed.

Let's first explore how it can show up in insight-oriented psychodynamic therapy. When someone is feeling insecure in their attachment to their therapist and does not know how to talk about it, they can, as Peter Fonagy said, "do crazy things" [5]. You can probably recall patients who seemed totally fine in their weekly sessions, until you went on vacation—and then all bets were off. Suicidal threats, calls in crisis in the middle of the night, and other intrusions during time off can generate anger, confusion, and resentment in the minds of most therapists. The therapist who is on vacation—usually a model of calm, cool, and collective Zen-like wisdom—is suddenly irritable and complaining to their partner that they want to fire the patient when they return from vacation. In this scenario, neither the therapist nor the patient is likely to be mentalizing well.

This teleological scenario is so common that the classic comedy *What About Bob* takes it to a rather extreme teleological boundary crossing. In that movie, a psychiatrist's nervous and insecurely attached patient, Bob, follows him and his family to his country house and ingratiates himself with the psychiatrist's family. Ultimately, this leads to the psychiatrist going insane. This movie came out in 1991, pre dating the development of mentalization-based treatment. What could he have done? We recommend that therapists caught in a teleological trap first validate the individual's wish for proof, without actually providing the proof, if it can be helped. Next, move on to naming the "elephant in the room" that this search for proof is problematic and address this shared dilemma head on. John Gunderson, in his model for generalist therapy for borderline personality disorder, was widely quoted as telling patients who would reach out in this prove-it mode that "You don't want your safety to depend on the likes of me!" [6]. He would, at the same time as naming that dilemma, validate how hard it is to feel that it does depend on the reaction of someone they care about, and make this dilemma a core focus of the work. Asking the patient what they would do in the therapist's shoes can be a game changer in getting mentalization going, as they usually have become so focused on getting a desired response that they lose sight that the therapist is a human with their own thoughts and feelings.

Teleological mode can wreak havoc on all therapy modalities if left unnoticed and unchecked. For example, in skills-based therapy such as DBT, therapists can sometimes get stuck in making themselves too available to their patients. Even the most conscientious DBT skills coach will miss an important phone call or text from a patient in crisis. They may emerge from an underground subway to a series of frantic texts culminating in the therapist being fired for not caring, accompanied by an image of the patient self-injuring, with the caption "THIS IS YOUR FAULT!!!" When they calm down several hours later, they send a message recanting the abrupt firing but still are angry that their therapist cared so little about them that they deliberately chose to ignore the call. The patient of course is not mentalizing and is certain that given that the therapist failed to provide proof they cared by answering the phone promptly, the therapist must have done so intentionally. Where it gets interesting from a mentalization standpoint is that the caring and responsible therapist may then feel guilty for letting their patient down and even though their supervisor assures them it is not their fault, the therapist feels compelled to make it up to the patient somehow. Maybe they offer an extra session. Maybe they decide they cannot ever take the subway again, so as to not miss another call. Whatever they do to prove that they do indeed care is an example of the therapist getting stuck in the teleological mode of interaction. We have all been there, and it is human nature to want to prove to others that we do in fact care. It is our contention that therapists will burn out very fast if they fail to recognize this teleological dead end. This may be one of the reasons why DBT consultation teams often include each team member rating their own burnout level at the start of each weekly meeting. One of the most valuable aspects of a well-run DBT program is the consultation team. As we have repeatedly said, working with patients who are suicidal or using NSSI, you must not act as a lone mentalizing ninja; instead, you must work collectively in a mentalizing social network of care (for you and the patient).

Finally, seeing mentalization as a skill to help people generate and maintain epistemic trust, so they can more effectively learn new skills rather than maintaining that their current perspective is the only right one, maps very nicely onto the DBT concept of *Wise Mind*. In DBT, therapists work to help individuals get into Wise Mind, where neither thoughts nor feelings dominate and instead work in harmony to inform one's perspective and maximize effective behaviors. In MBT, therapists work to help individuals get and keep mentalization online, where thoughts and feelings also work in harmony to broaden one's perspective and improve one's interactions in the world—"Holding the Balance." The goals are remarkably similar despite the different terminology. If one is in Wise Mind, one is likely mentalizing. If one is stuck in Emotion Mind, an MBT therapist would be on the lookout for psychic equivalence and teleological modes. If one is stuck in Rational Mind, an MBT therapist would be on the lookout for pretend mode, which can be highly intellectualized and divorced from feeling. Many DBT skills, such as the GIVE skill, are essentially cheat codes toward fostering mentalization and getting individuals into a Wise Mind state. GIVE is an interpersonal effectiveness skill that instructs someone who is trying to maintain a relationship to "be gentle, act interested, validate, and use an easy manner." This is remarkably similar to the mentalizing stance, is it not, dear reader?

Conclusion

Hopefully, through the above examples, we have convinced you that MBT really does "play well with others." It is no wonder that at trainings we attend, therapists from across the world—many with radically different therapeutic leanings—seem to find something fundamental about mentalization that resonates with their work and, in particular, with some of their more challenging cases. As we have discussed throughout this book, grappling with suicidal thinking and self-injury tends to send mentalization offline for therapists who start to worry about medico legal risks, feelings of limited control, and the need to face high levels of chaotic distress. Being armed with the knowledge that this is normal even for the most masterful expert in their respective therapeutic discipline, and that mentalization techniques can help the therapist get back into their groove, so to speak, is hopefully encouraging for you as you take the next steps in your therapeutic career.

References

1. Fonagy P. Are mentalization-based treatments old wine in new bottles? Presented at the Mentalization-Based Treatment 4th International Conference—Clinical Applications of MBT; London; 7–8 Dec 2017.
2. Allen JG. Handbook of mentalization-based treatment. Chichester: Wiley; 2006.
3. Fonagy P, Allison E. The role of mentalizing and epistemic trust in the therapeutic relationship. Psychotherapy. 2014;51(3):372–80.
4. Weitz E, Kleiboer A, Van Straten A, Cuijpers P. The effects of psychotherapy for depression on anxiety symptoms: a meta-analysis. Psychol Med. 2018 Oct;48(13):2140–52.
5. BorderlinerNotes. Peter Fonagy—the therapeutic effects of talking about thoughts & feelings. YouTube. https://youtu.be/OsYczfyOty0. Accessed 19 Jul 2019.
6. Gunderson J. Good psychiatric management (GPM) for borderline personality disorder (BPD): what every psychiatrist should know. Presented at the 2015 Oslo Conference; Oslo; 3 Dec 2015.

Mentalizing Crisis Management of Suicide and Self-Injurious Behavior

8

Owen Muir

Introduction

In this chapter, our goals are to help you consider how to actualize the mentalizing concepts laid out in the first five chapters in the midst of a crisis. Throughout this chapter we encourage you to actively reflect on several important concepts: what the active ingredients that allow mentalizing to occur are, what the mentalizing stance is, and how to intervene during the three most common pre-mentalizing modes: psychic equivalence, teleological mode, and pretend mode.

Dr. Jon Allen, from the Menninger Clinic, has a now-famous quote that is, in our team's collective minds, a perfect guide for this chapter. The quote, importantly enough, came from a patient with whom he was engaged in therapy. It reads, "The mind can be a scary place—you wouldn't want to go in there alone!" This chapter, along with Chap. 6, should make it abundantly clear that working with people who struggle with suicide and self-injurious acts requires a team. You are not, dear reader, a "mentalizing ninja," and you should be on alert for processes that may push you away from teams and disclosure of the challenges faced when young people are suicidal. Even outside training to be a therapist, a therapist always needs a mentalizing mind assisting them and their patient in order to help make sense of things that AREN'T MAKING SENSE.

This chapter is therefore a guide for using mentalizing in the midst of one of the scariest concepts in mental health: a patient who is *actively focused* on dying or engaging in self-injurious behaviors.

This chapter will discuss the following:

1. Mentalizing overview of suicide and non-suicidal self-injury (NSSI) crisis
2. Mentalizing young people who are actively suicidal or NSSI
3. Mentalizing young people after a suicide or NSSI act

O. Muir (✉)
Brooklyn Minds Psychiatry, Brooklyn, NY, USA
e-mail: Owen.muir@brooklynminds.com

L. L. Williams, O. Muir (eds.), *Adolescent Suicide and Self-Injury*,
https://doi.org/10.1007/978-3-030-42875-4_8

4. Effectively using supervision within a mentalizing frame
5. Mentalizing and a completed suicide—what comes next

Mentalizing Overview

The management of youth with chronic suicidality or NSSI, using mentalization-based treatment (MBT) for adolescents, offers guidance for how to deal with acute crisis situations that are often counter to traditional and prescriptive approaches. As with all things MBT, the core approach to a crisis is the "not-knowing" stance. Youth and families in crisis are often very sure that what is happening, whatever it is, is a CRISIS. The ability to stay "online" and be curious will help keep the nerves of any MBT practitioner a little calmer and the emotional temperature a little cooler, which gives you and the youth and families a chance to restore mentalizing.

To start, it's worth recognizing that crisis situations are an inherent problem for a mentalizing approach, as there is likely an increased emotional temperature from the patient, the family, or YOU, which makes mentalizing harder for everyone. Furthermore, in a crisis, typically everyone (the patient, the family, the emergency room (ER) physician, the school, YOU) expects "something" to be done, which can be quite teleological and possibly mindless.

These crises can be extremely challenging given that when to consider a higher level of care is most often the "something" that everyone is wanting or dreading, depending on who you are talking to. This means that careful consideration of the various clinical markers will be critical to taking the next steps treatment-wise. The research in this regard has something of a split mind. On the one hand, once a person has attempted suicide, their risk of future attempts is immediately higher, usually in the following two years, for both attempts and completed suicide.[1] However, individuals who repeatedly attempt suicide do not 100% of the time complete suicide, so risk factors that are temporal in nature are generally most important when considering the most immediate RISK of another attempt. This information is also generally true of those who self-injure. National studies on youth who partake in NSSI indicate that a higher percentage of youth try NSSI between one and three times, but only a small percentage of youth continue to utilize NSSI as a chronic strategy for emotional distress.[2] There are also data showing that youth who use NSSI are, at times, actively suicidal and NSSI places a person at higher risk of attempting suicide.[3] Importantly, there have been no randomized controlled trials to support the use of acute hospitalization in saving lives, but in cases of high acuity because of temporal risk factors or clearly abnormal mental states, hospitalization is

[1] Parra-Uribe I, Blasco-Fontecilla H, Garcia-Parés G, Martínez-Naval L, Valero-Coppin O, Cebrià-Meca A, Oquendo MA, Palao-Vidal D. Risk of re-attempts and suicide death after a suicide attempt: a survival analysis. BMC Psychiatr. 2017;17(1):163.

[2] Barrocas AL, Hankin BL, Young JF, Abela JR. Rates of nonsuicidal self-injury in youth: age, sex, and behavioral methods in a community sample. Pediatrics. 2012;130(1):39–45.

[3] Muehlenkamp JJ, Gutierrez PM. Risk for suicide attempts among adolescents who engage in non-suicidal self-injury. Archiv Suicide Res. 2007;11(1):69–82.

commonly undertaken. "Contracts for safety" have not been proven to be effective.[4] However, research has told us that a simple connection with a health team professional after the attempt (within 72 hours) decreases future suicide and NSSI acts.[5] In determining the level of active acute risk, a clinician can use a few evidence-informed screening devices: the Columbia Suicide Severity Rating Scale (C-SSRS),[6] the Linehan Risk Management and Assessment Protocol (LRAMP),[7] and the Ask Suicide-Screening Questions (ASQ) toolkit.[8]

Furthermore, the most crucial "suicide management" resource, in keeping with the MBT model, is other colleagues to help you think when emotions predictably run hot in the context of working with suicidal youth. Especially at more junior levels of training, you are likely to have a supervisor officially assigned, and likely several more informal mentors who you can and should turn to for assistance in holding onto your own mind in the context of high levels of anxiety around the potential death of a person you are working with. Remember Dr. Allen's patient and the axiom "Never worry alone."

Most models built for working with chronically suicidal individuals include some form of support. Dialectical behavior therapy (DBT) has the consultation team. MBT has *Thinking Together*, which is outlined in Chap. 6. In the MBT context, it is often helpful to keep at least one team member uninvolved in every case, so that someone can be as far away, mentally, from the mentalizing–collapsing chaos of the patient's difficulties. Frequently, multiple clinicians will be involved in the cases of high-risk patients and families, and rightly so.

To put it simply, if you are worried about a suicidal patient, and no one else knows about it, you are quite likely "doing it wrong." Turn to a colleague and document it! In summary, our goal in discussing mentalizing while in crisis is to more accurately understand the current situation such that a shared treatment plan can be conceptualized. We are not stating that mentalizing in a vacuum will prevent suicide or NSSI, but more that mentalizing can lessen the risks of suicidal or NSSI actions as a young person gains improved mentalizing skills in addition to their mentalizing socially connected team, of which you and your team are a part. Furthermore, we encourage therapists to recognize that you can't always pick your patients. If you are in the youth mental health field, you will have patients who become suicidal or turn to NSSI for relief. Having a grounded method for the approach to care with young people experiencing suicide or NSSI will help you "keep the balance."

---

[4] Drew BL. Self-harm behavior and no-suicide contracting in psychiatric inpatient settings. Archiv Psychiatr Nurs. 2001;15(3):99–106.

[5] Welu TC. A follow-up program for suicide attempters: evaluation of effectiveness. Suicide Life Threat Behav. 1977;7(1):17–20. https://onlinelibrary.wiley.com/doi/full/10.1111/j.1943-278X.1977.tb00886.

[6] Posner K, Brent D, Lucas C, Gould M, Stanley B, Brown G, Fisher P, Zelazny J, Burke A, Oquendo M, Mann J. Columbia-Suicide Severity Rating Scale (C-SSRS). New York: Columbia University Medical Center; 2008.

[7] Linehan MM. Linehan Risk Assessment and Management Protocol (LRAMP). Seattle: Linehan MM, 2014.

[8] Horowitz LM, Bridge JA, Teach SJ, Ballard E, Klima J, Rosenstein DL, Wharff EA, Ginnis K, Cannon E, Joshi P. Ask Suicide-Screening Questions (ASQ): a brief instrument for the pediatric emergency department. Archiv Pediatr Adolesc Med. 2012;166(12):1170–6.

Mentalizing Young People Who Are Actively Suicidal or Using NSSI

First, a brief note: although this approach is intended for both suicide and self-injury, we will use the term *suicidal* for brevity, though readers should understand that this applies to both NSSI and suicidal ideation.

First, for most clinicians, the worst thing that can happen as a helping professional is to lose a patient to suicide. This outcome strikes at the core of our own senses of agency and efficacy in the world, and makes us doubt everything about ourselves and our abilities. The loss of often unbelievably intimate relationships, even professional ones, is devastating. So much rides on suicide not happening that it is somewhat of a paradox that a mentalizing approach to this problem is even possible for THERAPISTS, much less adolescent patients. Working with suicidal youth is a bit like being a high-wire walker who is afraid of heights. We are always looking at our worst fear, and that puts our ability to mentalize in jeopardy.

Second, crisis situations pull helping professionals into "I'm a professional,"—and thus pretend mode. These "canned" questions and responses lead to saying things that are perceived as untrustworthy and not genuine. There is a good reason for this: they are often deeply phony! "I can contract for safety" is a phrase I hope none of us has uttered when out at brunch with family or colleagues. We don't say things like that for a good reason: they are usually as insincere and lacking genuine concern as they appear.

Third, crisis situations often end up involving more individuals and systems than just the client and the therapist. This can lead to predictable systems disintegration and generate further mistrust: "You said I was just going for an evaluation, and now they are admitting me to The Worst Hospital." As such, the decision to escalate to a higher level of care may be driven as much by policies and procedures to satisfy medicolegal requirements and thus aren't particularly flexible. For more on this concept, read Chap. 6 again even more carefully.

The "Not-Knowing" Stance in a Suicidal Crisis

However, dear reader, our radical concept is that *most crisis situations are actually a perfect fit for the mentalizing stance; almost axiomatically, if you "knew" what to do, it wouldn't be understood as a crisis*. Thus, genuinely accepting that you "don't know exactly what to do here" with your patients is a *first-line intervention*. The not-knowing stance that works for our patients to alleviate their distress is the same tool we have at our disposal, and luckily it works very well.

The Next Steps: To Paraphrase from the Classic Novel *The House of God*—A Few Guidelines

In a suicidal crisis, the first procedure is to take your own pulse.
—Samuel Shem, *The House of God*

Keeping our own mentalizing stance is the only prerequisite for effectively applying mentalizing therapy. It follows that all of the interventions that will keep our patients out of any of the three modes of pre-mentalizing thinking will do much the same for us. To further borrow from Samuel Shem's classic novel:

> The delivery of good medical care is to do as much nothing as possible.

That is to say, in this case, action is less useful than curious pauses. Clearly, doing "all nothing" isn't appropriate—that would be teleological in its own right. However, an entirely action-based plan is also ill advised and likely to be non-mentalized. Axiomatically, mentalizing needs to get back online in order for therapists and their patients to understand the crisis. So "Am I mentalizing now?" has to always be the first question we answer in responding to suicidal crisis moments.

Almost all suicidal moments are non-mentalized. So the second question we need to answer as a mentalizing therapist—"Is my patient mentalizing?"—has been answered for us already (finally, something easy). And the answer is "Nope."

Now, we get to the point of talking to the adolescent. Finally, some therapy can happen! Using our skills from Chap. 2, we have all the tools we need to get some mentalizing sparked. And that, as with all things mentalizing, is the magic—you don't have to solve whatever problem inspired the mentalizing collapse that led to the suicidal crisis in the first place. All we are here to do is help mentalizing come back online for the youth—and perhaps for others involved in the crisis response. Once someone is mentalizing, they almost, by definition, don't need to teleologically murder themselves, and thoughtful plans can be co-constructed (Fig. 8.1).

The following case vignette will feature first a more generic approach to a suicidal crisis. In the text in parentheses, our team is commenting on the likely pre-mentalizing modes of thinking by both the patient and therapist. Our goal here is not to belittle any specific approach to therapy, nor do we wish to have the therapist or the patient portrayed as "the worst." Our desire with this vignette is to ask you, dear reader, to consider two questions: (1) is either person mentalizing; and (2) if not, what type of pre-mentalizing mode is either person in?

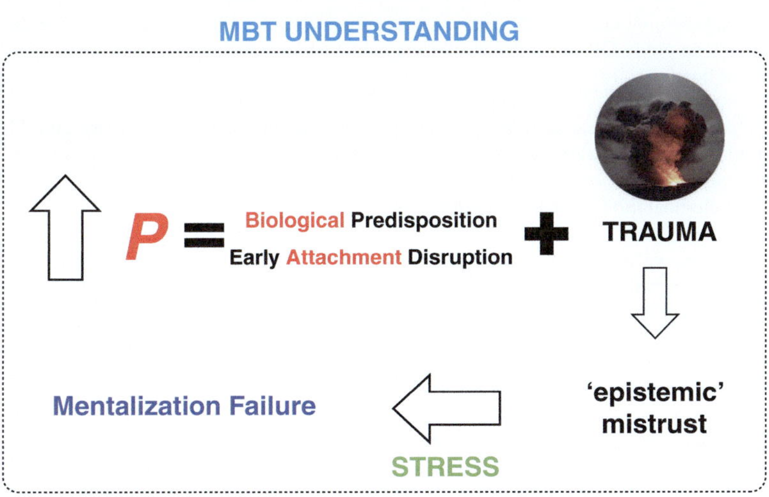

Fig. 8.1 Mentalization-based treatment (MBT) understanding. *P* psychopathology

Vignette

Jennifer's therapist is speaking at a conference next week. Jennifer is a 16-year-old with a history of obsessive–compulsive disorder (OCD), major depressive disorder (MDD), a mixed personality disorder with borderline and obsessive–compulsive personality disorder (OCPD) traits, posttraumatic stress disorder (PTSD), and a history of three suicide attempts and three subsequent hospitalizations, although none within the last year. She is quite intelligent and can alternate between being confident and outspoken and being fragile and in an almost dissociative state during therapy.

Presession

It is Friday, two days before the therapist is leaving town, and Jennifer sends frantic text messages in the morning, indicating that she is feeling even more suicidal and is afraid she will overdose on her clomipramine. She insists on meeting the therapist at the end of Friday to "solve it!" (teleological mode). Amazingly, the therapist has an open time at 4:30 p.m. that evening. During the phone call setting up the appointment, Jennifer says:

"Just don't go to your conference, and I'll be fine."
(Psychic equivalence)

Session

"Hey, Dr. M, I'm not OK with you leaving."
(Psychic equivalence)

"Why don't you back up and tell me what's happened since we last met?"
(Attempt to reframe)

"Aren't you listening? I think I'm going to kill myself if you go to that conference!"
(Psychic equivalence)

"I am listening, but I wasn't sure what had changed since our last meeting when things seemed to be going OK."
(Clarification)

"Things would be easier if you'd just give me your cell phone number. We could have dealt with this by text already since *obviously things are not going OK* [said sarcastically]. That is easier for me than waiting to see you."
(Teleological mode and some pretend mode)

"Jennifer, we've talked about my out-of-session boundaries before. I can't help but notice that you bring this up whenever you're upset with me. What do you think?"
(Pretend mode, likely because the therapist can't think of what else to say)

"NO ONE MEETS MY NEEDS EVER, DR. M!"
(Psychic equivalence: "EVER")

"Hey, Jennifer, let's try to calm down; maybe we can try the five-senses skill."
(Pretend mode of the therapist in response to psychic equivalence: iatrogenic)

"F*CK THIS! I'm gonna kill myself."
(Predictable enough, teleological mode)

"Can you tell me more? I'm trying to understand. Maybe we can map out with our screener the best next steps."
(Clarification attempts followed by panic at this point moves the therapist into teleological mode)

"NOT THAT STUPID SCALE AGAIN! I just don't want you to go. Then you will be far away, and what if bad things happen? WHAT IF, DR. M? WHAT IF?"
(Non-mentalizing at the start, BUT the patient has given the therapist a hint about how they feel)

"Look we've talked before about really being thorough when a safety concern comes up."
(Be careful with the word "look." It almost always comes across as condescending and is likely a flag for non-mentalized discourse and teleological mode on the part of the therapist.)

"I'm not threatening. I'm contracting to KMS if you go on vacation."
(More teleological mode; the therapist missed a window of mentalizing)

"I'd prefer it if we can work on a safety plan here that starts with answering these questions."
(Invalidating and in pretend mode; it feels more like it's in the therapist's best interests.)

"I NEED YOU HERE!"
(Plea for attachment and psychic equivalence)

"Jennifer, I have an idea: why don't you just leave your extra clomipramine with me? You can trust me to hang on to it, and then I won't have to worry about you overdosing."
(Teleological mode mixed with some pretend mode for good measure)

"I don't want to," the patient replies, and then stares at the therapist in silence.

"Jennifer…" says the therapist [in an exasperated tone].

"NO!" exclaims the patient. "I don't WANT to."

"Oh...well…"

Mentalizing the Moment

So what are the answers to the above questions? Is anyone mentalizing? Not really, although the patient got close a few times. What pre-mentalizing modes were occurring? For the patient, there was primarily the "hot" mode and for the therapist, the "cold" mode (pretend). As you can see in this typical interaction, the "hotter" the patient gets, the "colder" the therapist gets. Recall from Chap. 2 the concept of elasticity versus flexibility. Here the therapist has started off giving the patient an extra session (albeit for a good clinical reason) and quickly wants to move into "therapy problem-solving mode" but gets increasing distressed themselves as the patient keeps talking about suicide. Suddenly, the therapist snaps back with a teleological solution—"hold the medications"—even though neither person really understands yet what is actually going on.

Remember that Non-mentalizing Begets Non-mentalizing

Each person in the room, on some level, is protecting themselves as best they know how. Unfortunately, this protection is leading them both further away from actually understanding.

Now remember the first rule: check your own pulse and decide "AM I mentalizing?"

Let's say that this therapist has begun to recognize the coercive pattern occurring here. This allows us to reiterate the next most salient point: *mentalizing failures occur all the time, AND that is OK.* Own it with humility and humor, and work to get the mentalizing engaged again for you and the patient. You don't need to start over with a "perfect session" or a "clever thing to say." We are not recruiting mentalizing ninjas, we are asking you to re-engage in the NOT-KNOWING STANCE.

You will notice that the therapist doesn't quite know what to say, which we saw in Chap. 2 was a good way to tell that you might be dealing with the "feelings = facts" (non-mentalizing) mode of psychic equivalence. Even the thought "I'm stuck and don't know what to say" can be the start of your road map.

Session

"Jennifer, sorry! I really f∗#ed up here, didn't I?"
(Humility and practicing not knowing)

"Uh? What do you mean?"
(Confusion)

"You came in today because something was really upsetting you, and somehow I jumped ahead and started solving a problem I didn't understand. But I do want to understand."
(Clarification)

"Um, OK."
(Confusion)

"Can I get a do-over here, if you would be so kind, dear maiden? [said in a fussy formal voice] *Please tell me*: what's going on? [said in an earnest voice with more direct eye contact]"
(Rebuilding epistemic trust with MARKED mirroring)

[Laughs] "Dr. M, you are sooo weird."
(Humor re-engaged, emotions are cooling off, mentalizing is coming back online)

"So… [said in a fussy formal voice again]."

"Well, I told you I feel so hopeless, like I'm not going to EVER get better. What if I feel even worse while you're gone? I feel like I'm gonna die if I can't talk to you; that's why I want to be able to text you. You're the only one who gets me—ya know?"

(Mixture of psychic equivalence, but the tone of the conversation suggests a more open stance)

"Wow that's a lot to unpack, but I like that we're now both thinking together about this BIG problem of NEVER EVER getting better. That sounds like a really scary thought. Is it?"

(Validation mixed with some challenge)

As you can see, as the session progresses, both patient and therapist are more engaged with each other. Hopefully, the therapist can keep holding the balance as they learn more about the crisis and discuss a plan. Remember, this plan may even include having the medication secured more safely; it may include using the five-senses skill; it may include engaging more people from this young person's social network. These activities can all be part of mentalizing therapy, as the goal of mentalizing therapy is to mentalize. As we are understood by each other and ourselves, we are better able to incorporate new information, and learn and incorporate a meaningful plan of care.

Mentalizing Young People After a Suicide or NSSI Act

While MBT can be thought of as formal psychotherapy to be practiced according to a specific model, the core of mentalizing is that taking a not-knowing stance toward interpersonal interactions is vital regardless of your location of care. If thought of as a way of being trustworthy, built on a foundation of curiosity and genuineness, then mentalizing fits into any number of settings, including the emergency room (ER), where clinicians frequently encounter patients who have recently self-injured or already attempted suicide.

As a young clinician in an ER, I marveled at the "magic" my supervisor had in interacting with the sickest of patients. What I didn't realize then was that the magic had very little to do with how much she knew about various psychotropics or the variety of psychiatric disorders; it had more to do with her basic kindness and desire to "understand and be helpful." While I ran around frantically, gathering all the facts, I missed the first piece, or the lynch pin: really working to mentalize the other person. It's easy to miss when so much is coming at you, dear reader, but our advice to you, time and time again, is to pause and consider the question "Am I mentalizing myself and my patient?"

The behavioral emergency setting is one in which the accuracy of information is crucial in decision-making, and the ability to establish trust quickly is the difference perhaps between life and death. Often, especially with "involuntary" admissions, patients are brought in a highly mistrust-inducing way to the hospital, sometimes even in handcuffs! To begin a relationship, even a brief one, when one party is in the process of having their freedom taken away is often fraught with difficulty. Patients—especially those who have been in this situation before—often do not trust mental health professionals. Frankly, why should they? In the emergency room, the skill set of a therapist has been repurposed to determine if a patient will keep or lose their freedom. Clinicians also don't trust patients—they have every reason to try to want to mislead us in order to leave! Patients don't trust clinicians—they "just" want to lock them up! A more fraught environment for epistemic *mistrust* is hard to find.

But mentalizing is built on some core assumptions that can be helpful, even here in the ER.

First is the understanding that pre-mentalizing modes exist and are adaptive in some circumstances. Furthermore, in order to deceive another, it takes a misuse of mentalizing (generally in pretend mode) in order to "selfishly" but accurately hold the mind of another in mind well enough to make up a story that will be believable in that other person's mind.

Second, when mentalizing is restored, it becomes harder to stay in the kind of state where you can't imagine genuine benevolent intent on the part of the clinician. Simply, even the most difficult "frequent flier" will, if feeling understood and with mentalizing ability restored, be better able to imagine that a clinician actually might want to help, and thus it might be worth disclosing their actual needs.

Thus, all the skills you learned in the previous chapters in this book can be put to use in the ER for perhaps even more important ends than providing effective psychotherapy.

Third, a key to an accurate evaluation and good clinical decision making is being told the truth, as the patient understands it. And taking a curious stance is a fabulous way of generating trust; being *actually* interested in a patient's struggles can be a challenge all by itself given the frequently "phony" or pretend interactions that can happen in emergency settings.

When evaluating patients who have engaged in self-harm, the ability to generate epistemic trust via mentalizing interventions and a not-knowing stance is lifesaving. In practice, these are the steps you learned about in Chap. 2. Below is another case vignette highlighting first a non-mentalizing approach to a post-suicide ER visit, which then shifts to a more mentalizing interaction.

Vignette

A clinician approaches a young person lying in a hospital bed with a nasogastric tube inserted through their nose and gauze on their left wrist. They were admitted due to "swallowing some of their mother's pills and cutting the left wrist" after seeing an Instagram post from their ex-girlfriend late last night.

> "Hi, I'm Dr. M. The ER team told me you took some pills last night to try to die. Can we talk about that for a bit?"
>
> (Somewhat curious approach by the clinician, but pretty abrupt)
>
> "Can't I just sleep? [big yawn] I already told that other doctor I'm fine. Ain't no big deal."
>
> (This may be true fatigue, but pretend mode may also be activated)

"Sorry, no, we need to get this done now before you get admitted upstairs."
(Pretend mode; no curiosity, movement toward teleological mode)

"What? [now fully awake and irritated] I told you and those other people I am fine; I don't need any psycho ward stay. I have a big math test today."
(Pretend mode along with psychic equivalence)

"It seems hard to believe you are fine given that your Tylenol level is very high. Do you realize you could have died?"
(Lecture mode, i.e., pretend mode; still no curiosity toward the patient)

"Whatever—do what you want, I'm going back to sleep. This place sucks [mumbling and head turned away]."

Unsure what to do, since repeated attempts to communicate falter, the clinician walks away after saying they will talk with the family and come back. The clinician leaves the room—an active mentalizing approach that is sometimes needed—to regroup and consider what has just happened.

As a side note, recognizing pretend mode is an essential skill in a suicidal crisis:

> A key is to recognize that mixed non-mentalizing states can be happening in suicidal youth. There is the stereotype that suicidal means "too hot" emotionally. This is often, but not always, true. Many suicide attempts, especially in those with personality pathology, occur in pretend mode.
>
> Pretend mode, again, is a state in which the attachment activation is too low and the emotions are too cold. Words and feelings don't match. It's the land of "whatever" and "I don't know" responses. In this state, patients become disconnected from their internal experience to a marked degree, and this sense of emptiness feels awful. To profoundly "not at all" have words for how one feels is difficult, but on a scale that only suicidal youth and infants are routinely familiar with. People can get so disconnected that the "only way" (as suggested by their failure of mentalizing) to understand how they feel might be to attempt suicide or self-harm. Once one has sliced one's wrist, it's hard to mistake what happened, and the attempt becomes the proof of how the person MUST have felt. "I must be suicidal—I tried to kill myself." This is, of course, the definition of another non-mentalizing mode: teleological mode. The action taken—a suicide attempt—determines the internal state. "I was suicidal, and I know this cause my wrists are bleeding."

The clinician returns as the nurse is taking vital signs and chatting with the young person.

"I see you're awake; how are you feeling? I imagine that tube in your nose is irritating; has the team explained to you what it's for?"
(Curious, attempting to validate a possible feeling the patient may be having)

"I guess, sorta; they said it had to do with my liver or something, I dunno really."
(Pretend)

"You're right; it is about your liver. I can tell you more if you like, but I also wanted to talk some more about what happened; d'you remember me, that annoying doctor from the psycho ward?"
(Validation, humor, a small challenge to raise the temperature)

"Sure; I don't need to go to any psycho ward, like I said."
(Communicating at least)

"Well, the thing is, I don't know either—that's actually one of the main reasons I wanted to talk with you. Can we chat for a bit?"
(Validation without agreement, an invitation to be curious)

"I guess—nothing really to say; I told you nothing's wrong. The picture just surprised me, is all. I'm over it now."
(Wow, all over the place, but maybe a nugget of feeling there)

"Could be, could be, but still, it did seem pretty surprising from what you are saying. Maybe tell me a bit more about it, and we could figure this out?"
(Using patient word choice, validation again without agreement, more curiosity as the patient is beginning to engage)

As you can see in the above vignette, the use of the mentalizing stance, paying attention to the emotional temperature, and then activating maneuvers to engage once a patient is in a specific pre-mentalizing mode can clearly assist a clinician to work to gather an honest clinical picture after a suicide attempt. It is our contention that imbuing the work you do with mentalizing does not make your processes longer (indeed, it may short-cut explosive outbursts or walls of silence) and ultimately it will be more accurate and compassionate. Again, depending on the total picture, this young person may need admission, but even then you can start the admission off in a more hopeful place that allows for engagement.

Effectively Using Supervision Within a Mentalizing Frame

Often, a clinician managing a crisis in the community setting will do so by phone or text messaging. This section will focus on crisis phone and text interactions, and how they can be used to manage crises as they arise in the lives of clients.

First, a note about intersession contact and availability: many health systems make this difficult to do. Working with suicidal adolescents and their families without judicious use of intersession contact is not an approach that we would recommend. How you manage that availability will likely become part of the therapeutic work. However, in order to really understand suicidal youths' difficulties in the moment, and being able to intervene in crisis, it is our shared opinion that a mentalizing therapist and their team needs availability outside office hours.

We urge you to engage with the health care system you are working with as it relates to preferred HIPPA (Health Insurance Portability and Accountability Act)–compliant modes of communication, as that is beyond the scope of this book. The decision to "be available" should be a decision that is planned out in advance and in accordance with policies and an appropriate structure for you and the patient. If you are dealing with someone who is a danger to themselves, expect your mentalizing to go offline from time to time. Simply put, if you have read this book this far, having ongoing supervision is a lifelong recommendation!

Supervision in Real Time: Texts and Phone Calls in a Crisis

The example below is one such team arrangement. In Chap. 6, there is a great section on the specific reasons for a proscribed mentalizing supervision approach that is slightly different than the one offered below. We would recommend that you discuss both types of supervisory approach with your team of teams so that the scope and purpose are clear from the outset.

The following is a text example of one of our clinicians interacting with a suicidal client and receiving supervision in the actual moment of a patient crisis (with the details changed to protect their identity):

Clinician: "How're you doing?"

Youth: "In bed, crying, I have so many memories that are bad"

Clinician: "Would it help to do one of the occupying headspace things we talked about?"

Youth: "I don't know"

Clinician [after an hour's pause]: "Did you give it a try in the end? I apologize for being in and out, I want to be present, but at the same time I'm pretty busy today"

Youth: [texts a picture of a handwritten suicide note]

Clinician: "Claire?"

Clinician: [in an internal communication to the medical director and clinical director for supervision] "Need Help Here"

Clinician: "Please respond and let me know you are still here"

[Pause of several minutes]

Youth: "I came outside with my dog, I wanted to walk her"

Clinical director: [in an internal communication] "My heart just started beating again…was typing to call 911 if there was radio silence after THAT note"

Clinician: "I am glad you took your dog out for a walk. Holy shit, I was scared for a minute there!"

Clinical director: [in an internal communication] "Seriously!"

Clinician: [in an internal communication] "My next patient was here already and I was about to have a panic attack"

Clinical director: [in an internal communication] "I mean she really seems to be upping the ante as of late and it is very scary to bear witness and not be able to do much to stop it other than try to connect with her as you are doing. I worry with every rehearsal or half-hearted attempt she gets more acclimated to following through"

Clinician: [in an internal communication] "Yes, that is for sure a concern. I think some of it is maybe trying to force me to reject her because at least part of her actually does trust me and that might be terrifying, both because I could use it to hurt her and because if you have something you could lose it…if that makes sense?"

Clinical director: [in an internal communication] "Yes"

Clinician: [in an internal communication] "Do you think it's useful for me to say that? Perhaps in conjunction with the thing you said about it being scary to bear witness to it and not be able to do much to stop it?"

Clinical director: [in an internal communication] "Yeah I think if she is engaged and somewhat mentalizing that might work—otherwise I don't think it will really register"

Clinician: [in an internal communication] "I think I may try tomorrow unless she messages again tonight"

[End of crisis supervision]

Mentalizing and a Completed Suicide—What Comes Next

The Worst Has Happened—Understanding and Coping with Patient Suicide

I'll begin with an introduction from a piece by Sulome Anderson, which I turned to for guidance after the death of my patient. It featured her friend who was, at the time of this interview, admitted to a specialized inpatient unit:

> "I completely fell apart after my therapist quit, because I relied on her very heavily," she says. "I got really attached to her, and it's so hard when someone you care about, that you trust, decides not to work with you anymore. It makes you feel like they think you're never going to get better. It felt like she gave up on me."
>
> I ask her if she knows why she can't find another doctor who will take her on as a patient, and she sighs.
>
> "Because I take up so many more resources than other patients," she says. "I tried calling people from *Psychology Today*—you know how they have those listings? They're nice at first, but when I tell them how suicidal I've been, all of a sudden, they don't really have time, and they don't know anybody they can refer you to ... nobody wants to work with someone like me. It's a risk, because if we do kill ourselves, it's traumatizing and messes them up. And also, they can get sued." [1]

My patient (who I will call "Phil" here) was discharged from a hospital into the care of our mentalizing team, which included an individual therapist, a physician to manage his medical regime [this author], and groups. In the year that followed, with a relentless focus on improving mentalizing for the patient, a remarkable relationship unfolded, and a remarkable person began to live his life in the world, not in the confines of the hospitals and residential programs he had spent the prior decade of his life in. He returned to inpatient psychiatry only once, for a planned titration of medication.

For a year, his ability to be in the world with family, friends, and work blossomed. However, the obsessions with suicide returned, and he spent a night in the ER. I visited the next morning, spoke to the resident on call, and spoke extensively to the father and patient. We devised a relatively simple safety plan, which included a scheduled visit for medication management the following day.

He was discharged home. I got a phone call at 6 p.m. (one of the thousands of such calls I'd received) which felt more hopeful: "I don't want to kill myself, but I feel like I have to."

Later that night, not having heard from Phil again, the therapist took the unusual step of calling our patient. The phone was turned off.

The next morning, while in my own individual therapy session, I received a phone call from the patient's father. I picked it up on speaker.

"Phil is dead.... He is dead," his father mumbled.

The world kept spinning, but with one less remarkable soul in it, and the grief began for all those who knew him, and continues from time to time to haunt all of us who knew Phil.

As the readers of a book on working with suicidal youth, you are part of an audience that recognizes that there is risk in the patients we work with.

That death has had a profound effect on me. It is not, given my current field of specialty, my only loss to suicide, nor will I expect them to cease. Yet, at the same time, I continue to engage with young people who are feeling suicidal. I feel that I must, but I recognize that in order to do this work honestly and well, I must continue to be supported by a mentalizing team around me.

What do we know about physicians and therapists coping—or struggling—with patient suicide? After all, the death of a patient from severe illness is not foreign to the field of medicine. No oncologist has the expectation that all of their patients will survive stage 5 cancer. Trauma surgeons do their best, and yet still sometimes the injuries will be too severe. We have morbidity and mortality conferences to discuss bad outcomes and learn lessons as a fundamental part of being in this profession. Yet, suicide is understood differently from other deaths. Perhaps this is due to the stigma still attached to mental health and illness; perhaps it is due to the fear of contagion. Much remains to be understood about suicide.

After losing a patient to suicide, a complex process of grief and trauma will unfold. With support and trust from those in our mentalizing circle, it can resolve. Below is a helpful structure to consider when a suicide occurs.

1. If in training, call your program director immediately for support.
2. Call your supervisor and/or mentalizing team as soon as is reasonable for support.
3. If you have completed your training, call your malpractice carrier. This is important, and they will have useful things to say. In training, your program director will likely assist you, as the case will involve a supervising clinician and system of care with their own legal team.
4. Unless specifically told not to by your malpractice carrier or training program, reach out to the family and offer your thoughts and support.
5. If possible, attend the funeral. This is hard, but it's unlikely you will regret it.
6. Check in with your therapist (if applicable) promptly.
7. Schedule time with your team to discuss the case.
8. Don't go into the chart to fix or improve any aspect of the care. If a final encounter or appointment had not yet been documented, discuss with your program director and legal team how best to complete the documentation.
9. Don't (in the immediate period afterwards) endlessly review notes or things you could have done differently. It is natural (and nothing we could write would convince you otherwise) to review your documentation. But leave the deep dive to your malpractice carrier if they choose to do that.
10. Plan to be sad. Go home from work as soon as you can logistically do so, and while staying connected to colleagues. Strongly consider some time off from work. The most useful question I was asked by a supervisor at work after losing Phil was "Why are you here?" Lacking a compelling answer, I went home.
11. Don't isolate yourself.
12. As hard as it is to accept, as someone reading a book about working with suicidal and self-harming youth, you are highly likely to have patients end their

life in ways you could not prevent. *Your willingness to work with suicidal youth will, however, likely save the lives of countless more and, unlike each suicide, each choice to live won't be known to you much of the time.*

Conclusion

Suicide and non-suicidal self-injury are scary. Remember, though, that it is scary for your patients and their families as well; in fact, they are probably more scared than you. Treatment can be successful, especially in a team-based setting. While you can do your best to screen patients, the fact remains that for a clinician who is considering working with youth, suicide and non-suicidal self-injury will occur. The mentalizing skills learned through this book, and specifically this chapter, may better prepare you and your mentalizing teams (the patients, and yours) to assist young people toward a path of recovery through enhanced mentalizing. As we said at the outset, "The mind can be a scary place—and you wouldn't want to go in there alone!"

Reference

1. Anderson S. How patient suicide affects psychiatrists. The Atlantic https://www.theatlantic.com/health/archive/2015/01/how-patient-suicide-affects-psychiatrists/384563/. Accessed July 2019.

Mentalization-Based Treatment for Adolescents: The Framework for Work with Suicide and Self-Injurious Behaviors

9

Trudie Rossouw, Owen Muir, and Laurel L. Williams

Introduction

In this chapter, our focus will be to pull from the previous chapters the necessary building blocks for mentalization-based treatment for adolescents (MBT-A). This chapter will lay out the MBT-A framework to further highlight both the metaprocesses involved in using mentalizing as a theoretical model of and the specific techniques and tasks, modeling for you, dear reader, the outline—or "manual"—for MBT-A.

At the end of this chapter, the reader should be able to:

1. Identify why mentalizing is the focus for treatment of suicidal and self-injurious youth
2. Identify the mentalizing assessment process
3. Identify the elements of a mentalizing formulation
4. Identify the specific procedural elements in MBT-A

A Recap: Why Is Mentalizing the Focus for Suicidal and Self-Injurious Youth?

Hopefully, over the course of this book, a strong case has been laid out as to why this very specific concept of "seeing yourself from the outside and seeing others from the inside" is the core of treatment efficacy. If therapy were done via

T. Rossouw
Priory Hospital North London, London, UK

O. Muir
Brooklyn Minds Psychiatry, Brooklyn, NY, USA

L. L. Williams (✉)
Menninger Department of Psychiatry and Behavioral Sciences, Baylor College of Medicine, Houston, TX, USA
e-mail: laurelw@bcm.edu

L. L. Williams, O. Muir (eds.), *Adolescent Suicide and Self-Injury*,
https://doi.org/10.1007/978-3-030-42875-4_9

internet-connected apps on your phone, mentalizing would be the 5G wireless signal that allows the apps to communicate and function. In MBT-A, we focus on the concept that mentalizing is a core human trait and a necessary skill to be able to learn a wide variety of knowledge. Once more, people can't learn how to make their lives better if they aren't "online" with their mentalizing. It's as basic as not being able to log on to Facebook (for your adolescents, that will be Snapchat) if there is no reception! Mentalizing is also the path to being interpersonally effective. We have discussed the pre-mentalizing modes of thinking (psychic equivalence, teleological mode, and pretend mode) that hopefully give way to a "balanced stance" and that as a therapist you have been introduced to techniques that can help restore mentalizing in yourself, the young person, their family, and maybe a system of care you have joined with. We have reviewed how mentalizing impacts families and how you can engage in mentalizing work beyond the young person. We have furthermore reviewed with you how a wide variety of mental health challenges or disorders are impacted by mentalizing (both positively and negatively). We have thoroughly discussed how using mentalization can be lifesaving in moments of suicidal and self-injurious crises, even outside a formal psychotherapeutic relationship. We have additionally discussed the fact that the system's "default setting" is disintegration and that as a mentalizing therapist it would be wise to be engaged in a team approach to this care or, at the very least, to be well versed in how social connections and systems can enhance or inhibit mentalization. Finally, we have discussed how mentalizing is congruent with most forms of psychotherapy.

From our perspective, our task in MBT-A therapy, broadly, is to help the young person get back on the right "developmental track." This includes helping kids and families achieve a sense of autonomy, identity, and eventually mastery. Once they can keep a mental model of minds handy, they will be more able to have more realistic experiences both by themselves and with others. Mentalizing ends the interpersonal confusion and makes both kids and families resilient.

To study the hypothesis that mentalizing improvements—the goal of MBT-A—improve the lives of troubled youth, our colleagues ran a prospective study of 150 young people who were admitted to an adolescent unit. Hauser et al. found at 10-year follow-up that a surprising number of these young people performed in the top half of all adults in terms of social and emotional functioning [1]. Hauser et al. identified three main protecting factors in the high-performing group, which were as follows [1]:

- A capacity for reflection about their own thoughts, feelings, and motivations
- A sense of agency—i.e., a sense of oneself as effective and responsible for one's actions
- Relatedness—an ability to reflect on the minds of others

In other words, the protective factors that helped these youth excel could be summed up as a capacity to mentalize. This capacity to reflect upon their own internal state and; the mind of the other, and their sense of responsibility about themselves and the impact they have on the minds of those around them, were the unifying factors in good outcomes later in life [2, 3]. This was borne out in the first MBT-A randomized controlled trial run by Rossouw and Fonagy [4], in which young people with suicidal and self-injurious behavior randomly received MBT-A or cognitive behavioral therapy (CBT) over the course of one year. While both groups did see improvements, the MBT-A group not only had improvements in the target behaviors (self-injury (SI) and non-suicidal self-injury (NSSI)), but also saw enhanced social connectedness and a decrease in depressive symptoms in comparison with a well-managed CBT treatment program.

In MBT-A therapy, our aim is to increase the ability to be mindful of oneself and those around one in a more accurate way—as well as being mindful of the impact one has on others. In achieving greater and more accurate awareness about the minds of others, impulsive behavior will reduce and hence risk will reduce. This too will reduce the storminess of relationships that is so typical in the absence of mentalization. This leads to more stability in life. A stable life leads to a sense of hope as well as mastery over the things kids have to do every day. If it seems like a big sell—"This one ability makes everything better!"—be assured, dear readers, that we see it every day! Mentalizing is the 5G of interpersonal effectiveness.

In MBT-A, parents and kids are enlisted to work as partners in a treatment designed to shift from discussing *behaviors* (that doubtless need to *stop*) to a mentalizing conversation that enables family members to grasp each other's point of view and share their own in a palatable way. Shifting away from trying to force change helps rekindle curiosity, respect, empathy, mutuality, and agency in a family. We unabashedly are teaching kids and families how to be MBT therapists in their own right!

As we discussed in Chap. 3, coercive and non-mentalizing cycles in families are unlikely to change without active intervention. Thus, the aim of MBT-A is to help families shift from coercive interactions to mentalizing ones that can promote trust and secure attachment. To do this, we need to limit the parent's experience of incompetence in treatment. As we discussed in Chap. 3, caregivers can't feel blamed or shamed for their children's problems, or therapy won't generate the epistemic trust needed (remember that the airplane oxygen mask needs to be placed on the ADULT first). Similarly, young people need to feel more understood by others and themselves. Without trust, mentalizing therapy (or any other type of therapy) will not work.

At times you may be pulled to feel more aligned with the young person than, say, the father. If the father begins to feel that his mind is not being kept in mind, the treatment can wither on the vine. Allowing for multiple perspectives can be challenging to hold in one therapist's mind. This is why having a team can give voice to each person's unique strengths and challenges, so if local resources allow for a team approach, dear reader, create a mentalizing team. Use the information from Chap. 6 to map out who is either the "structural hole" (we really need a better term, don't we?), or a "weak dyad" that needs a connector to become a triad, which, as you will recall, is a more stable setting that encourages mentalizing to flourish. Remember, since we don't expect you to be a lone mentalizing ninja, recognize that sometimes the weak link is you—the therapist—and, as such, you need your mentalizing bolstered by a team member.

Adolescents are faced with the developmental task of building a sense of autonomy and personal identity. However, they often feel themselves overwhelmed by experiences of failure. Their experiences can be a sea of bewilderment in dealing with others or with relationships, often leading to a sense of helplessness and self-hatred. They often wish to "just" give up. (Remember that in MBT-A, the word "just" is literally and metaphorically a four-letter word.) Frequently, when we see these young people, they have dropped out of their social world—and sometimes have even dropped out of school—and have given up any hope that they can achieve anything in their lives. Their interpersonal relationships fill them with anxiety and fear. They worry that they will be rejected or that they are not liked. They spend a great deal of time "overthinking" the intentions of others. This leads to a state of mental anguish, which fuels self-hatred. Very soon, the suffering can no longer be endured and they respond with impulsive behavior, such as self-harm in order to "get rid of" the pain. They become avoidant and can "skip" school or are embroiled in drama-heavy interpersonal relationships. These relationships swing between over-involvement and avoidance of intimacy in close relationships. Their lives resemble a cruelly curated reality show, full of chaos, and they reliably become involved with similarly disturbed characters who gravitate to the same ill-advised activities. BUT don't forget the parents (caretakers), because, as we discussed in Chap. 1, the four attachment styles are often passed down INTERGENERATIONALLY, meaning that how the young person is feeling and acting may actually have a great deal of continuity with the experiences of the adults, if the adults are given space for their minds to be understood as well.

Assessing Mentalizing

If, dear reader, you start to work and breathe in a mentalizing place, your assessment process will fuse with mentalizing. This may be a bit cheeky, but we ask you to concretely consider, for a moment, "What is the goal of an assessment?"

Have you thought about it? We'll give you a few minutes more. [Cue the *Jeopardy* theme music.]

We imagine that came up with quite a number of items. The following are a few feeble attempts to consider what might be in your mind:

1. To assess mental states
2. To assess for safety
3. To make a diagnosis
4. To develop a treatment plan

These are all great things, and we have little doubt that you likely came up with an even longer list, but the point here is that *as you MENTALIZE WITH THE PERSON/FAMILY while asking about all of the above,* you are getting, IN REAL TIME, how the young person or family mentalizes. We ask you to ADD this information into your formulation. Throughout this book, there are numerous examples showing how to pull for more mentalization, but if we leave you with nothing else, we hope that you are able to recall that BEING CURIOUS and practicing the "NOT-KNOWING" STANCE are ESSENTIAL. What is essential? Being curious and the not-knowing stance. Why is that repeated? We mentalized you, dear reader, and wanted to make sure that even if you glazed over when reading the first sentence, the planned redundancy of the second would help drive the point home. We strongly encourage you to use these mentalizing tools while meeting with a young person and their family during your assessment process (Box 9.1).

Box 9.1 Systems of care issues

Our understanding is that everyone has different system constraints when it comes to both the *how* and the *when* of assessments, as well as the type and cadence of sessions after the assessment. Part of a mentalizing stance for us is to be cognizant that adaptation to your local system of care will likely be necessary. Our promise to you, dear reader, is that the more you incorporate mentalizing into your therapy headspace, the richer and better informed your assessments and treatments will become.

So often, young people who are chronically suicidal or using NSSI are caught in a frightening inner world of self-hatred, which renders them vulnerable to expecting similar feelings of disdain from the world around them. They often shut themselves off from the world around them, as they already "know" what people are feeling and thinking about them. In the authors' experience, these youngsters often relate to themselves in a dehumanizing way. Remember, "dehumanized" is a non-mentalized view of a human and allows self-harm or violence against the non-person the young person finds themselves to be. It is essential for us to embody humanity in our interactions with young people in therapy. We show authentic interest and curiosity about the young person's life and mind, and we explore the richness of all possibilities in a non-judgemental way. Active questioning expresses curiosity; it should be expected to yield not an unequivocal answer but progress toward a conceptualization of alternatives [5].

In the situations where young people harm themselves, it is at times hard for family members and helping professionals to remain empathic and warm. Family and staff can often feel that self-inflicting injuries are deliberately "treatment interfering" or attention seeking. Parents and staff can feel undermined, angry, powerless, or very anxious. Not uncommonly, parents and staff can at times feel that "You are doing this deliberately to make me feel powerless or anxious" (psychic equivalence happens to us all in moments of extreme stress).

Parents and staff can be helped to develop greater understanding and less hostility by getting to know that self-harm in young people is hardly ever done for the purposes of "seeking attention"; instead, it is done as a desperate way to try and cope with unbearable feelings inside them. We also challenge you to consider "What is going on for this young person?" if they actually are "doing it for attention." How does that make sense? Until those feelings have been understood and individuals have developed greater abilities to mentalize, it is our contention that those states of dysregulation are likely to reoccur.

Adopting the core mentalizing not-knowing stance allows us to ask many questions, such as "What happened before you felt like hurting yourself?" Remember that mentalizing therapy is active. We do not adopt a neutral stance, nor do we allow for long silences. This is particularly helpful when young people find it hard to relate to their inner worlds. An example would be a young person who says, "I *just* felt like cutting myself; it was *just* an overwhelming urge that came into my mind. It has no other meaning" or "Nothing happened before I felt like that." The not-knowing stance means we do not know what that feels like and it leaves us with a desire and a curiosity to get to know more. Hence, we would ask questions in order to try and learn more about the young person's experience. We may say, "Tell me a little bit more about what you were doing before you felt like that…where were you…or what were you thinking…or, if I was a fly on the wall, what would I have seen?" The message is "I really want to know what you experienced; take me there so we can look at it together." This stance is about getting to know the patient's experience and, in that process, the feelings will unfold themselves and this will make it easier to explore or make emotional contact with the affect.

In summary, for the young people and their families you are working with, a mentalizing assessment that actively uses the mentalizing stance is key [6]:

- An ability to communicate with the patient in a direct, authentic, transparent manner, using simple and unambiguous statements so as to minimize the risk of overarousing the client
- An ability to adopt a not-knowing stance, which communicates to the patient a genuine attempt to find out about their mental experience
- An ability to sustain an active, non-judgmental mentalizing stance that prioritizes the joint exploration of the patient's mental states
- An ability to communicate genuine curiosity about the patient's mental states by actively enquiring about interpersonal processes and their connection with the patient's mental states
- An ability to follow shifts and changes in the patient's understanding of their own and others' thoughts and feelings
- An ability to become aware of and respond sensitively to sudden and dramatic failures of mentalization in the patient

Elements of a Mentalizing Formulation

As you complete your assessment of the young person and their family, we encourage you to develop a formulation of their mentalizing capacities. This should hopefully be a bit familiar, as we practiced formulation with Lydia and her family in Chap. 3. In this formulation you are considering the strengths and vulnerabilities of each person and also, as we discussed in Chap. 6, the strengths and vulnerabilities of the systems that the young person and family find themselves in. The goal here is to create a counderstanding that will evolve over the course of treatment. Indeed, if, at the end of therapy, the final formulation were to look identical to the initial formulation, this would seem to support the idea that (a) therapy is not yet complete yet, or (b) what was the purpose of the formulation or therapy to begin with?!

For MBT-A, a formulation is meant to be "alive." As we discussed in Chap. 3, we actively use the verb *mentalizing* versus the noun *mentalization*. As you reflect on what you have learned about the mentalizing capacities of the young person and their support team, you model bringing this to them in a session where you invite everyone to make improvements to the formulation and coconstruct the mentalizing action plan.

Formulation Example

"Thanks everyone for coming in today for a joint session. I want to start off by saying how much I have enjoyed getting to learn more about each of you. [Here, insert something brief that you have learned about each person in the room that connects to mentalizing.] I can see both the warmth and the strong desire to be in a better place, as well as the pain each person is feeling given the current challenges. My hope here today is to discuss with you how we can take this information and use it to craft a treatment plan that moves us toward a better understanding of our misunderstandings. Remember that funny word I have brought up a few times: "mentalization"? Well, this funny word is actually a powerful tool we can all use to make change. The good news, as I have said before, is that everyone in the family already does mentalize, but what happens is that there are times where mentalizing goes offline. The hard part is that it can go offline at different times and for different reasons for each person. So a big goal for us will be helping to recognize when it goes offline and what skills we will all need to improve to get it running again. We will start out doing these tasks together, but over time the goal is for you to each be able to do this for yourselves individually and also, maybe even more importantly, collectively. We say "collectively", because what we know about this idea is that everyone needs help sometimes in getting mentalizing back online. Think of me as your tech support, in that I am going to help teach you how to get it back online without me. Pretty cool stuff, yeah? What do you think; can that be something we work on together?"

Structure of MBT-A

MBT-A is usually combined with MBT-F (MBT for Families) and MBT-G (MBT for Groups). It includes the following stages of therapy:

- The assessment (1–3 sessions)
  - Building a therapeutic relationship
  - Safety plan
  - Formulation

- The bulk of the work (6–8 sessions)
  - Improving mentalizing and impulse control
  - Enhancing awareness of the mental states of others
  - Help with adolescent tasks
- The final phase (3–4 sessions)
  - Increasing independence and responsibility
  - Consolidating stability
  - Developing follow-up plans
  - Understanding and processing the meaning of the ending, with a focus on affective states associated with loss
  - Discharge and liaison with partner organizations

So, dear reader, what do you think of this MBT-A structure? I mostly suspect there is a big fat YAWN at this point. I have a bit of trepidation to confess to you, dear reader, if you were to ask me to do a brain scan, as I worry that you were hoping for something more dramatic or "new." But the reality is that this structure should not at all seem new. The story of humankind is always done in threes. You might call this the TRILOGY OF MENTALIZING [intoned in a Gandalf-ingly EPIC voice]. First, you get introduced and connected to the young person and their family, as well as to the mentalizing challenges, and consider your mentalizing road map. Then you actively work on these challenges, through a great deal of active mentalizing, stopping coercive cycles and creating named mentalizing loops that allow for continuity between sessions. Finally, you assist in generalizing these changes so that you say good-bye to an important and meaningful human connection. Remember, as we discussed at the end of Chap. 3, we consider that this is not THE END; instead:

> What we are shooting for is more than a happy ending. It's a curious series of endings, over and over again, with each understood misunderstanding making the next more likely!

It is beyond the scope of this chapter to describe the phases in great detail, but much of what has been discussed in the previous chapters should allow you to see how to use this structure in mentalizing therapy. Again, as we imagine you, dear reader, we can see you go "Wait!"—your brow furrows and your emotions get a bit hotter—"Hey, what about suicide or self-harm? I don't see anything about that VERY IMPORTANT issue in that very boring mentalizing trilogy" [thinking to yourself, "I never liked Gandalf that much"].

Dear reader, WE COMPLETELY AGREE WITH YOU [looking directly into your eyes for some mirrored marked contingency]: self-harm and suicide ARE IMPORTANT. Thank you for telling us how you are feeling in the moment. We do want to give you more concrete information about MBT-A management of self-harm and suicide. We agree and believe it would be extremely helpful to discuss the safety plan, which should be drawn up with young people as early on in therapy as possible. The aim of the safety plan is to give young people and their families something concrete to guide and help them in between sessions; ultimately, it is a plan to keep the young person safe and to upskill the family to keep the young person safe.

We do the safety planning in two stages if the individual therapist and family therapist are not the same person. However, we recommend that by the end of the safety planning, there is only one "plan," which everyone has contributed to. We also expect (or maybe HOPE is a better word) that the safety plan is updated as therapy progresses. This is much like the formulation we have discussed on numerous occasions; as understanding improves across the family, there is likely refinement and nuance added to the plan.

Stage 1: The Family

The crisis plan with the parents includes education for them on our basic understanding of self-harm and risk in young people, with practical advice on how to behave and what to say/do when young people self-harm. It also includes advice on basic safety measures at home to reduce the risk.

"As a parent we want to protect our children from harm because it brings up strong feelings such as helplessness, anxiety, anger, frustration, and fear. We hope that this crisis plan will give you some guidance at the start of treatment. We hope to see this plan improve as we learn together what works best as we strive to improve how your child and family are doing."

Step 1: Basic Safety Measures

- Keep medications locked away, including over-the-counter medications. Safely remove old prescriptions from the home and consider purchasing medications in smaller total doses (instead of a 100-tablet bottle, consider a 25-tablet bottle).
- Remove weapons from the home or, at a minimum, have weapons safely secured (in a lockbox) and stored separately from ammunition.
- If your child harms themselves by cutting themselves, it may be helpful if you keep the knives out of reach, including restricting access to razors.
- It may also be helpful if you remove "sharps" from your child's bedroom.
- Ask your child if there are other items around the house that they fear they may use to self-harm.

Step 2: Guidelines for Communication About Self-Harm

We strongly recommend you consider how to be able to "hear" that your child feels at risk of self-harm or suicide. Since we know that this is a main focus for treatment, we expect to talk even more about how to help you and your child during therapy, but of this beginning time we strongly encourage the following:

Recognize that young people will find this very hard to do. Below are some ways to make it easier:

- Use a "safe" word for danger.
- Texting "I'm unsafe" or using predetermined emoji may be easier than talking.

If your child is very much at risk:

- Be with them as well as considering who may be best suited to assist in this manner (ensure the person is an adult and is aware that they are serving in this capacity).
- Sometimes you need to sleep in the same room as your child.

Young people mostly harm themselves when they have very strong feelings inside them that they find hard to manage. Here are several dos and don'ts that may help you at times of risk:

Dos:

- Do listen curiously.
- Do attempt to understand.
- Do let them know you are there for them.

Don'ts:

- Don't panic.
- Don't blame or shame.
- Don't punish.
- Don't use hospitalization as a threat or punishment.

Try to not blame your child, and try harder to not blame yourself. Instead, try to understand what your child felt before they wanted to harm themselves and help them to speak about the feelings and the events leading up to those feelings. If the events involved you, listen and try to understand their perspective—but don't become defensive, or catch yourself if you do!

You don't have to hold the same perspective, but it is important that you validate their perspective. If there was a misunderstanding between you that you contributed to, own up to it. *Remember, you are here not to win battles with your child but to restore the connection between you.*

If your child is very upset, speaking too much is not helpful. Just be kind and supportive, and say things like "I am not angry with you, I am here to help you and keep you safe. Something has made you so upset. I don't know what it is and if it is something I have done, I am sorry. We can talk more when you are ready."

If your child wants to hurt themselves, you could say, "I really don't want you to hurt yourself. I can see from [XYZ] that you said hurting yourself makes some sense to you…so maybe we can try an alternative? I'll help you; shall we get a bowl of ice?"*

If your child is suicidal, you could say, "Killing yourself is not a great option. I love you and don't want you to kill yourself. Do you feel alone? I'm right here. We'll get through this together. I'm going to stay here with you to keep you safe. Let's try and think of something that will help right now. Will distraction help, such as going for a walk or watching TV? Is there anything else that you find helpful?"

---

*Ice diving or another TIP (temperature change, intensive exercise, and progressive relaxation) skill from dialectical behavior therapy (DBT) can be borrowed liberally! Remember we discussed that in mentalizing therapy we encourage cross-colonization of approaches.

If all else fails, call the clinic or, if it is after hours, you may have to take your child to the emergency room (ER).

The safety plan for young people covers the areas mentioned above, such as a discussion about safety measures and communication with their parents when they are at risk by using code words or emoji on their phones. Additionally, the aim of the safety plan is to provide them with some skills they can make use of as alternatives to self-harm. These are to a large degree drawn from DBT skills and from mindfulness, but in reality they should be activities or skills that the young person has indicated an interest in or already finds successful in reducing the intensity of their thoughts or feelings. The first author of this chapter (T.R.) has created a phone app called COPING SKILLS, which offers DBT distress tolerance skills, mindfulness techniques, and distraction techniques, as well as guided meditation. The app also has a mindfulness section, which helps the young person to stop and pause and explore the interpersonal world they are in from a mentalizing perspective.

Safety Planning

Here is an example from a young person's therapist reviewing information gathered to help inform the development of a safety plan:

Trigger factors that you and I identified are times when you feel rejected, humiliated, or bad about yourself. As we've discussed, these feelings don't just arrive out of the blue; they're likely to have been triggered during an interaction with another person. You've expressed to me that when you have those feelings, you tend to rush into an action to take the feelings away. You told me you aren't really sure yet that you want to stop self-harming, but you've agreed that there are some parts of self-harm that make your life harder. You also talked about a few things you do find helpful or you might be willing to try out if you find your emotions or thoughts are running toward ACTION!

When you feel like that again, I'd like you to try and stop the action by trying to delay it for 10 minutes. Then use the 10 minutes to try and reflect on what was happening a few moments before you had the bad feeling. That might help you to understand more clearly what it is that you feel, as well as what might have happened in a close relationship that may have contributed to the feeling. You have talked about how you like to write; maybe during that time, write out all the thoughts that are coming to you. Once you have this understanding more clearly, it may be easier to think about a solution or to see things from a different perspective. Once that has happened, you may not feel as if you need to rush into action anymore.

If that fails or you don't feel like sitting there with your thoughts, and the urge to ACT remains SUPER STRONG, maybe you can turn to music (anyone for a little Beyoncé and dancing to *All the Single Ladies*?) or other types of ACTION that can help your body "do something." You have talked about how you liked that breathing exercise we tried. Again, what we do here is a physical action to help distract you from the URGE to self-harm.

You also talked about how sometimes you self-harm when you're in a "fog" or a "daze", and you can't even remember cutting until after you see the blood.

Although it might be hard, try and bring yourself back to reality. Don't just sit and stare into space with your mind full of negative thoughts about yourself. Do you remember how we talked about having a rubber band on your wrist? When you feel like you're going into a daze, consider snapping it; that reminds me of that Eminem song where he says "Snap back to reality." Get yourself back to reality, and then you can use one of those above ACTIONS for distraction.
If all else fails, call the clinic and ask to speak to me, and I'll call you back when I can.

Hopefully, you can see that even an initial safety plan does start out with some basic education (laying out the mentalizing stance with the dos and don'ts) but should have some personalized elements even at the outset. It can be helpful if this plan is teleologically written out (teleological mode is not always bad!). As we discussed in Chap. 8, no one needs to sign this; it's not a contract (remember, contracts have not been found to work) but it can be the concrete beginnings of better planning, communication, and action when mentalizing inevitably goes offline and self-harm or suicidal thoughts surface.

Conclusion

Dear reader, you did it: you finished this book. Our mentalizing team is in awe of you. We hope that in reading this book, you discovered many ways in which you are already doing a GREAT JOB mentalizing. We also hope that you found some ways in which you can incorporate more mentalizing into the therapeutic work you engage in. Mentalizing is fundamentally a team sport, and we hope that our journey together has been successful. Let's worry together; it really does make therapy—and life—better.

References

1. Hauser ST, Allen JP, Golden E. Out of the woods: tales of resilient teens. Cambridge: Harvard University Press; 2006.
2. Bateman A, Fonagy P. Effectiveness of partial hospitalization in the treatment of borderline personality disorder: a randomized controlled trial. Am J Psychiatr. 1999;156:1563–9.
3. Bateman AW, Fonagy P. Psychotherapy for borderline personality disorder: mentalization based treatment. Oxford: Oxford University Press; 2004.
4. Rossouw TI, Fonagy P. Mentalization-based treatment for self-harm in adolescents: a randomized controlled trial. J Am Acad Child Adolesc Psychiat. 2012;51:12.
5. Skårderud F. Eating disorders. In: Bateman A, Fonagy P, editors. Handbook of mentalizing in mental health practice. Washington, DC: American Psychiatric Publishing; 2012. p. 347–84.
6. Anna Freud National Centre for Children and Families. Mentalization-based treatment for adolescence (MBT-A) training programme. https://www.annafreud.org/training/mentalization-based-treatment-training/mbt-a-training-programme/. Accessed 1 Dec 2019.

Index

L. L. Williams, O. Muir (eds.), *Adolescent Suicide and Self-Injury*,
https://doi.org/10.1007/978-3-030-42875-4

MIX
Papier aus verantwortungsvollen Quellen
Paper from responsible sources
FSC® C105338

If you have any concerns about our products,
you can contact us on
ProductSafety@springernature.com

In case Publisher is established outside the EU,
the EU authorized representative is:
Springer Nature Customer Service Center GmbH
Europaplatz 3, 69115 Heidelberg, Germany

Printed by Libri Plureos GmbH
in Hamburg, Germany